THE CARBOHYDRATE ADDICT'S CALORIE COUNTER

DR. RACHAEL F. HELLER
ASSISTANT PROFESSOR EMERITUS, MT. SINAI SCHOOL OF MEDICINE•
ASSISTANT PROFESSOR EMERITUS, GRADUATE CENTER OF THE
CITY UNIVERSITY OF NEW YORK

DR. RICHARD F. HELLER
PROFESSOR EMERITUS, MT. SINAI SCHOOL OF MEDICINE•
PROFESSOR EMERITUS, GRADUATE CENTER OF THE
CITY UNIVERSITY OF NEW YORK•
PROFESSOR EMERITUS, CITY UNIVERSITY OF NEW YORK

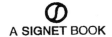

A SIGNET BOOK

A Note to the Reader
The ideas and data contained in this book are not intended as a substitute for medical treatment by a physician. The reader should regularly consult a physician in matters relating to health.

SIGNET
Published by New American Library, a division of
Penguin Putnam Inc., 375 Hudson Street,
New York, New York 10014, U.S.A.
Penguin Books Ltd, 27 Wrights Lane, London W8 5TZ, England
Penguin Books Australia Ltd, Ringwood, Victoria, Australia
Penguin Books Canada Ltd, 10 Alcorn Avenue, Toronto, Ontario, Canada M4V 3B2
Penguin Books (N.Z.) Ltd, 182–190 Wairau Road, Auckland 10, New Zealand

Penguin Books Ltd, Registered Offices
Harmondsworth, Middlesex, England

First published by Signet, an imprint of New American Library,
a division of Penguin Putnam Inc.

First Printing, January 2000
10 9 8 7 6 5 4 3 2 1

 REGISTERED TRADEMARK—MARCA REGISTRADA

Printed in the United States of America

**You are about to discover a
CALORIE COUNTER
like none you have ever seen!**

The 4000 food comparisons* in this counter are presented in two new and exciting reader-friendly formats.

Gone are the endless rows of tiny numbers that require the use of higher math and calculators before you can make a food choice.

A revolution in counters, these simple designs present food counts in clear, easy-to-read graphs that will make you exclaim, "Wow! Now I can see it all—at a glance!"

A-to-Z charts, found in the front of this counter, list foods in alphabetical order within several major categories. This format will help you to quickly and easily find a particular food by its name. Numbers at the end of each bar indicate specific caloric counts.

Hi-Low Comparison charts, found in the second half of this counter, rank foods from low to high. This format will help you to effortlessly select a "best choice" from any given category of foods. Again, numbers at the end of each bar indicate the specific caloric count.

All the Carbohydrate Addict's Counters give you the information you need to put you in control and to make gram and calorie counting exciting and fun!

*Nutritional values in this counter were taken from material supplied by or direct communication with the U.S. Department of Agriculture, scientific studies, computer data banks, and representatives of the food industry. When counts, as provided by a variety of sources, differ one from the other, an average or typical count is calculated and used. All data are rounded to the nearest whole number. Neither the authors nor publisher assume any responsibility for any errors contained herein and all readers must work in accordance with and in conjunction with their own personal physician. For information on abbreviations, see the introductory pages that follow.

CONTENTS

Introduction xi

| | Alphabetical Charts Begin | Hi-Low Comparison Charts Begin |

Beverages .... 2 .... 84 ....

Bread, Crackers, and Flours .... 5 .... 87 ....
    Bagels
    Biscuits, Rolls and Muffins
    Breads
    Crackers
    Dry and Crispy Foods
    Pancakes, Stuffing, and More

Cereals .... 11 .... 93 ....

Combined and Frozen Foods .... 17 .... 99 ....

Dairy .... 21 .... 103 ....
    Cheese (Hard and Semi-soft)
    Cheeses (Soft), Creams, and Substitutes
    Eggs, Milk, Yogurt, and Shakes

Dining Out .... 24 .... 106 ....
    Asian
    Delicatessen
    French and Other International Dishes
    Italian
    Mexican

Fast Food .... 29 .... 111 ....
    Arby's
    Boston Market
    Burger King
    Hardee's
    Jack in the Box

	Alphabetical Charts Begin	Hi-Low Comparison Charts Begin

Fast Food (*cont.*)
  KFC
  McDonald's
  Pizza Hut
  Subway
  Taco Bell
  Wendy's

Fruits ....40 ....122............
  Fresh and Dried Fruits and Juices

Gravies, Sauces, and Dips ....42 ....124............

Meats ....43 ....125............
  Beef
  Lamb
  Liver
  Pork
  Veal
  Other meats

Meats, Processed ....45 ....127............
  Beef jerky
  Bologna
  Chicken lunch meats
  Corned beef
  Ham
  Hot dogs
  Kielbasa
  Knockwurst
  Pastrami
  Roast beef
  Salami
  Sausage
  Turkey lunch meats and sausage

	Alphabetical Charts Begin	Hi-Low Comparison Charts Begin
Medications	46	128

Cough Drops and Syrups
Over-the-Counter Remedies and
    Vitamins and Minerals

| Miscellaneous Foods | 48 | 130 |

| Nuts, Beans, and Seeds | 49 | 131 |

| Oils and Fats | 51 | 133 |

| Pasta, Whole Grains, Rice, and Noodles | 52 | 134 |

| Poultry | 54 | 136 |

Capon
Chicken
Duck
Goose
Pheasant
Quail
Squab
Turkey

| Salad Bar Choices and Salad Dressings | 55 | 137 |

| Seafood | 57 | 139 |

| Snack Foods and Chips | 59 | 141 |

Cheez puffs
Chips, all varieties
Fruit rolls
Goldfish
Popcorn, all varieties
Pretzels
Rice cakes
Snack bars
Snack mixes

	Alphabetical Charts Begin	Hi-Low Comparison Charts Begin
Soup	61	143
Sweets	63	145

Cakes
Snack Cakes
Candy
Cookies
Donuts
Gum and Mints
Ice Cream
Ice Cream Cones, Bars, Alternatives, and Puddings
Pies and Snack Pies
Sugars, Syrups, Toppings and Jams

| Vegetables | 79 | 161 |
| Vegetarian Choices | 82 | 164 |

INTRODUCTION

Are You Addicted to Carbohydrates?

After breakfast, are you hungry before it's time for lunch? Once you start to eat breads and other starches, snack foods or sweets, do you have a very difficult time stopping? Do you snack when you're not really hungry? If so, it is likely that you are a carbohydrate addict. You may respond differently to that bread or pasta or potato, to those snack foods or sweets, than other people do.

Researchers have begun to confirm what many of us knew all along, that when it comes to eating and weight, as in so many other things, each of us is different. C. Everett Koop, M.D., the former Surgeon General of the United States, notes that some of us are "carbohydrate sensitive." As many as 75 percent of the overweight, and a good percentage of normal-weight individuals as well, appear to have a physical imbalance that leads to an addiction to carbohydrates.

Carbohydrate addiction is the result of an imbalance in the hormone insulin, and this "hunger hormone" makes us crave carbohydrate-rich foods intensely and repeatedly.

If you are addicted to carbohydrates, it is not your fault! Those of us who are carbohydrate addicts have genes that make us exceptionally good at storing carbohydrates in the form of fat. No matter how great our desire to stop eating and lose weight, our bodies seem to fight us at every level. Our basic constitution makes carbohydrate-rich foods taste exceptionally good and makes us more likely to put on weight and keep it on.

If you are addicted to carbohydrates, we hope you come to understand that carbohydrate addiction is not a matter of will-power but of biology. Your cravings and weight gain are symptoms of an underlying physical imbalance. We know what causes it and now we know how to correct it.

Carbohydrate addicts often find that:

- Once they start to eat bread, pasta, or other starches, snack foods or sweets, they have a difficult time stopping.
- After a full breakfast, they get hungry before lunch.
- They get tired and/or hungry in the mid-afternoon and a snack makes them feel better.
- They gain weight easily and/or, after dieting, tend to quickly gain weight back.
- They continue to eat or snack when they are not hungry.
- They sometimes lose control of their eating.

If, like so many others, you are addicted to carbohydrates, it is no mystery to us why you have struggled to stay on diet after diet, why diets often fail to help you keep the weight off, and why you may suffer from insulin-related health problems.

If you are a carbohydrate addict, starches, snack foods, junk foods and sweets may hold the key to your addiction and to your victory as well. On our Programs, you will find that you can enjoy these foods every day, in satisfying quantities.

For our Programs' essential guidelines, see *The Carbohydrate Addict's LifeSpan Program* (Plume), *The Carbohydrate Addict's Healthy for Life Plan* (Plume), *The Carbohydrate Addict's Diet* (Signet) or *The Carbohydrate Addict's Healthy Heart Program* (Ballantine). Our companion workbook, *The Carbohydrate Addict's Program for Success* (Plume), offers help with the emotional and spiritual aspects of carbohydrate addiction, and our other Carbohydrate Addict's Counters (Signet) can provide vital facts for success.

A Special Message from the Authors

Both of us were overweight children and adolescents. In time, as predicted, we became overweight adults. We grew up knowing the caloric content of foods as well as we knew the multiplication tables. And each of us, independently, struggled with calorie counters for as long as we can remember.

The calorie counters of three decades ago were uninteresting little books filled with columns of tiny numbers that were confusing to look at, difficult to read, and impossible to remember. After a tedious search for a food value, we easily forgot it by the next day. Comparing the calorie content of one food to another seemed to require the intelligence of a rocket scientist.

How could anyone be expected to compare ⅓ cup of one cereal with one ounce of another cereal? In some cases, milk and sugar were included, in other cases they were not.

As authors ourselves, we now understand that the writers who compiled these books included noncomparable quantities because doing so was a quick and easy way to take information directly from databases. In the past as now, we think this short-cutting does a terrible disservice to the reader.

Surprisingly, most of today's calorie counters do not look much different, nor are they any easier to use, than those counters of three decades ago. Many people have come to expect that calorie counting is a tedious necessity employed in the attainment of one's health and weight-loss goals.

We have found the opposite to be true and we think that you will too!

You are about to discover that calorie counting—and comparing—can be fun. In the Carbohydrate Addict's Counters, comparisons of calories, carbohydrates, and fats, respectively, become meaningful and easily understood.

In an instant you will be able to visualize the caloric contents of the entire aisle of cereals on your supermarket shelves. You will be able to intelligently choose the best meat for your weight-loss or health-related goals, and you will be able to select, with confidence, the dessert that is "worth" the calories. Fast food restaurants will now present a range of offerings, some of which will prove to be surprisingly better choices. The nutritional and caloric contents of meats, vegetables, snacks, sweets, and thousands of other foods become easy to grasp and hold in your mind.

Best of all, you will grow more confident with each success you achieve.

Between the two of us, we have lost over two hundred pounds, and we have maintained our ideal weights for over fifteen years. We are in perfect health for the first time in our lives, and our energy is unbounded.

We wish for you the permanent weight-loss and ideal health that we have achieved after so many years of struggle. The challenges of the past have made our present success that much sweeter.

What Is a Calorie?
Calories are used to measure the amount of energy stored in a food. All calories in food come from either carbohydrates, proteins, fats or alcohol.

How Many Calories Do I Need?
It was believed for many decades that the intake of 3,500 excess calories would result in a weight gain of one pound of fat. Likewise, it was assumed that reducing your caloric intake by 3,500 calories would bring about a one-pound loss of fat.

Recently, scientists have confirmed what most dieters have always known. When it comes to the impact of calories on weight gain, we are not all created equal. Two people can eat the same food and one will gain weight, while the other will lose weight. The way in which our bodies utilize calories is dependent on a wide variety of influences, including our genetics, lifestyle, muscle mass, activity level, age, gender, and a great deal more.

Primarily, the number of calories we need is determined by:

1. How Much Muscle We Have
Muscle mass has the greatest influence on caloric need. Eighty percent of the calories we burn come from our resting metabolic rate (calories burned while at rest), and much of our resting metabolic rate is directly related to how much muscle mass we have in our bodies. Increase your muscle "bank book" and, chances are, you will burn more calories.

2. How Much Total Weight We Carry Around

The heavier we are, even if the weight is extra body fat, the more energy our bodies need to move from point A to point B. As you lose weight, you may find that you reach weight-loss plateaus. One reason may be that your body doesn't need to put out as much energy to move you around.

3. How Far We Move Our Weight in a Day

The farther you move, the more energy you need. It's a simple fact of physics. Likewise, running burns more energy than walking for the same amount of time because running carries us farther. Like a car, if you go farther, you'll burn more fuel. You might be surprised to learn that running two miles burns only a slightly greater number of calories than walking two miles because you cover the same distance.

Given these variations, the best indicator of your ideal caloric intake is your own body fat level.

On the average, in order to maintain desirable weight, men need about 2,700 calories per day and women need about 2,000 calories per day. Each gram of fat contains about 9 calories; each gram of carbohydrate or protein contains about 4 calories.

It is not well understood why some people can eat much more than others and still maintain a desirable weight. However, one thing is certain: to lose weight, you must take in fewer calories than you burn. This means that you must either choose foods with fewer calories, or you must increase your physical activity—preferably both.

While only your physician can help you to determine the ideal caloric intake for you, here are some parameters that some health care professionals offer as a starting point.

From the left column of the chart that follows, choose the row closest to your current weight (or, if you like, the weight you would like to be). Moving to the right, find the column that best describes your activity level. In the box where these two intersect, you will find the approximate number of calories needed to support that weight level, assuming that activity level. Remember that individual differences can greatly influence this number, so take your knowledge of your body (as well as your physician's recommendations) into account.

If you now weigh or you would like to weigh	If you are sedentary, you should take in	If you are moderately active, you should take in	If you are very active, you should take in
100 lbs	1300 calories	1500 calories	1700 calories
125 lbs	1625 calories	1875 calories	2125 calories
150 lbs	1950 calories	2250 calories	2550 calories
175 lbs	2275 calories	2625 calories	2975 calories
200 lbs	2600 calories	3000 calories	3400 calories
225 lbs	2925 calories	3375 calories	3825 calories
250 lbs	3250 calories	3750 calories	4250 calories

How Much Should I Weigh? Three Tests to See If You're Overweight

Your height, age, muscle mass, and weight distribution all influence your weight and help determine the best weight for you. Physicians and researchers generally recommend three ways of determining your ideal weight.

Test #1: Weight Range Charts

The first way to determine your ideal weight is by consulting a published chart of desirable weights. The standardized chart on the following page is used by the United States Department of Agriculture.

Test #2: Pinch an Inch

While weight-range charts can help you to determine whether you have a weight problem, they cannot tell the whole story. Some people weigh more than the chart indicates to be "desirable," but their excess weight is primarily attributable to muscle mass. Others may find that they are not overweight according to the chart but are concerned that the placement of those extra pounds puts them in the "need to lose" category.

If you want to try a simple and quick test, pinch a fold of skin at the back of your upper arm. If you can pinch more than an inch, you are probably carrying more weight (in the form of fat) than is desirable.

RANGE OF "DESIRABLE" WEIGHTS*

Height without shoes	Weight without clothes	
	Men (pounds)	Women (pounds)
4'10"		92–121
4'11"		95–124
5'0"		98–127
5'1"	105–134	101–130
5'2"	108–137	104–134
5'3"	111–141	107–138
5'4"	114–145	110–142
5'5"	117–149	114–146
5'6"	121–154	118–150
5'7"	125–159	122–154
5'8"	129–163	126–159
5'9"	133–167	130–164
5'10"	137–172	134–169
5'11"	141–177	
6'0"	145–182	
6'1"	149–187	
6'2"	153–192	
6'3"	157–197	

*United States Department of Agriculture Human Nutrition Information Service Agriculture, Information Bulletin 364.

Test #3: Body Mass Index (BMI)

Most scientists and physicians have started to use Body Mass Index Scores as a way to get a better picture of an individual's weight level. Designed as a tool for statistical analysis, the BMI can help health professionals make evaluations regarding health risk factors related to excess weight.

Using a mathematical formula, the BMI takes into account both a person's weight and height. BMI equals a person's weight in kilograms divided by height in meters squared ($BMI = kg/m^2$). But don't worry, the table that follows will make it easy for you to get your BMI score.

To use the BMI table that follows, find your height (in inches) in the left-hand column. Move across the row to your weight. The number at the bottom of your weight column is your Body Mass Index (BMI).

BODY MASS INDEX CHART

Height (in.)

Height														
58	91	96	100	105	110	115	119	124	129	134	138	143	167	191
59	94	99	104	109	114	119	124	128	133	138	143	148	173	198
60	97	102	107	112	118	123	128	133	138	143	148	153	179	204
61	100	106	111	116	122	127	132	137	143	148	153	158	185	211
62	104	109	115	120	126	131	136	142	147	153	158	164	191	218
63	107	113	118	124	130	135	141	146	152	158	163	169	197	225
64	110	116	122	128	134	140	145	151	157	163	169	174	204	232
65	114	120	126	132	138	144	150	156	162	168	174	180	210	240
66	118	124	130	136	142	148	155	161	167	173	179	186	216	247
67	121	127	134	140	146	153	159	166	172	178	185	191	223	255
68	125	131	138	144	151	158	164	171	177	184	190	197	230	262
69	138	135	142	149	155	162	169	176	182	189	196	203	236	270
70	132	139	146	153	160	167	174	181	188	195	202	207	243	278
71	136	143	150	157	165	172	179	186	193	200	208	215	250	286
72	140	147	154	162	169	177	184	191	199	206	213	221	258	294
73	144	151	159	166	174	182	189	197	204	212	219	227	265	302
74	148	155	163	171	179	186	194	202	210	218	225	233	272	311
75	152	160	168	176	184	192	200	208	216	224	232	240	279	319
76	156	164	172	180	189	197	205	213	221	230	238	246	287	328
BMI (kg/m²)	19	20	21	22	23	24	25	26	27	28	29	30	35	40

Using your BMI score, the chart below can help you to better determine your weight level.

BMI (Body Mass Index)	Weight Assessment
18.5 or less	Underweight
18.5–24.9	Normal
25.0–29.9	Overweight
30.0–39.9	Obese
40 or greater	Extremely Obese

What This Book Can Do For You

All of the Carbohydrate Addict's Counters provide a whole new way of looking at food values—a simple and fun way to keep track of your eating and help you to make healthful choices.

We hope that this counter will become a good and well-used friend. It carries with it the experiences of over half a million people, along with our best wishes for a long, healthy, and happy life.

An Important Note

Any change in diet should be made in consultation with your physician. The data contained herein are not intended to re-place medical advice. Any questions or concerns should be addressed to your physician.

What Really Counts

Of all the important tools that are available to you, the most important by far is the commitment you bring to making your dreams come true.

So choose the best foods for you, plan and prepare healthful meals and, as appropriate, keep count of the calories you con-sume. In the counting, make certain to count on yourself—your strength, your love of life, and your desire to make your body and your life happy and healthy. You are your most important resource.

ABBREVIATIONS YOU'LL FIND IN
THE CARBOHYDRATE ADDICT'S COUNTERS

When You See This Abbreviation. . . .	It Means This
/	or
bl cheese	blue cheese
broc	broccoli
ch	cheese
dress	dressing
env	envelope
fl	fluid or flavor
flav	flavor(s)
Fr dress	French dressing
frzn	frozen
G'ma's Big	Grandma's Big
marg	margarine
parm	parmesan
Pepperidge	Pepperidge Farm
pkg	package
pkt	packet
q'tr pnd'r	quarter pounder
reg	regular
saus	sausage
Stella D	Stella D'Oro
sweet'd	sweetened
Thous Island	Thousand Island
tom	tomato
veg	vegetable
w/	with
wh	white

THE
CARBOHYDRATE
ADDICT'S
CALORIE
COUNTER

ALPHABETICAL CHARTS

BEVERAGES*, Part 1

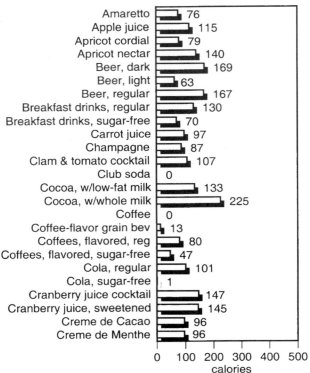

Beverage	Calories
Amaretto	76
Apple juice	115
Apricot cordial	79
Apricot nectar	140
Beer, dark	169
Beer, light	63
Beer, regular	167
Breakfast drinks, regular	130
Breakfast drinks, sugar-free	70
Carrot juice	97
Champagne	87
Clam & tomato cocktail	107
Club soda	0
Cocoa, w/low-fat milk	133
Cocoa, w/whole milk	225
Coffee	0
Coffee-flavor grain bev	13
Coffees, flavored, reg	80
Coffees, flavored, sugar-free	47
Cola, regular	101
Cola, sugar-free	1
Cranberry juice cocktail	147
Cranberry juice, sweetened	145
Creme de Cacao	96
Creme de Menthe	96

0   100   200   300   400   500
calories

* Counts for non-alcoholic drinks and beer are based on
8-fluid-ounce servings, for wine on 3 1/2-fluid-ounce
servings and, for hard liquor, on 1 1/2-fluid-ounce servings.

Alphabetical Chart
(for Hi-Low Comparison Charts, see pages 83 - 164)

BEVERAGES*, Part 2

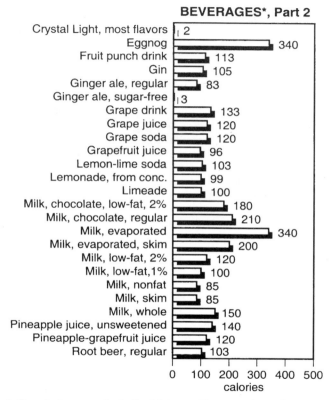

	calories
Crystal Light, most flavors	2
Eggnog	340
Fruit punch drink	113
Gin	105
Ginger ale, regular	83
Ginger ale, sugar-free	3
Grape drink	133
Grape juice	120
Grape soda	120
Grapefruit juice	96
Lemon-lime soda	103
Lemonade, from conc.	99
Limeade	100
Milk, chocolate, low-fat, 2%	180
Milk, chocolate, regular	210
Milk, evaporated	340
Milk, evaporated, skim	200
Milk, low-fat, 2%	120
Milk, low-fat,1%	100
Milk, nonfat	85
Milk, skim	85
Milk, whole	150
Pineapple juice, unsweetened	140
Pineapple-grapefruit juice	120
Root beer, regular	103

* Counts for non-alcoholic drinks and beer are based on
8-fluid-ounce servings, for wine on 3 1/2-fluid-ounce
servings and, for hard liquor, on 1 1/2-fluid-ounce servings.

BEVERAGES*, Part 3

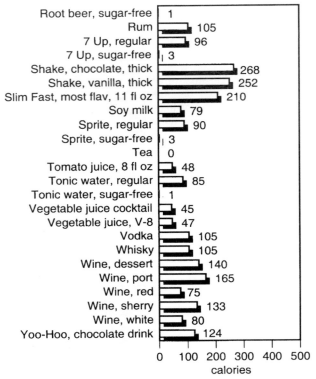

Beverage	calories
Root beer, sugar-free	1
Rum	105
7 Up, regular	96
7 Up, sugar-free	3
Shake, chocolate, thick	268
Shake, vanilla, thick	252
Slim Fast, most flav, 11 fl oz	210
Soy milk	79
Sprite, regular	90
Sprite, sugar-free	3
Tea	0
Tomato juice, 8 fl oz	48
Tonic water, regular	85
Tonic water, sugar-free	1
Vegetable juice cocktail	45
Vegetable juice, V-8	47
Vodka	105
Whisky	105
Wine, dessert	140
Wine, port	165
Wine, red	75
Wine, sherry	133
Wine, white	80
Yoo-Hoo, chocolate drink	124

0   100   200   300   400   500
calories

* Counts for non-alcoholic drinks and beer are based on
  8-fluid-ounce servings, for wine on 3 1/2-fluid-ounce
  servings and, for hard liquor, on 1 1/2-fluid-ounce servings.

4

Bread, Crackers, and Flours:
BAGELS*

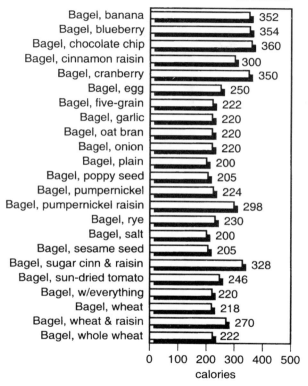

Bagel	calories
Bagel, banana	352
Bagel, blueberry	354
Bagel, chocolate chip	360
Bagel, cinnamon raisin	300
Bagel, cranberry	350
Bagel, egg	250
Bagel, five-grain	222
Bagel, garlic	220
Bagel, oat bran	220
Bagel, onion	220
Bagel, plain	200
Bagel, poppy seed	205
Bagel, pumpernickel	224
Bagel, pumpernickel raisin	298
Bagel, rye	230
Bagel, salt	200
Bagel, sesame seed	205
Bagel, sugar cinn & raisin	328
Bagel, sun-dried tomato	246
Bagel, w/everything	220
Bagel, wheat	218
Bagel, wheat & raisin	270
Bagel, whole wheat	222

0   100   200   300   400   500
calories

* Counts are based on one bagel, approximate weight:
  3 ounces.

Bread, Crackers, and Flours:
BISCUITS, ROLLS & MUFFINS*

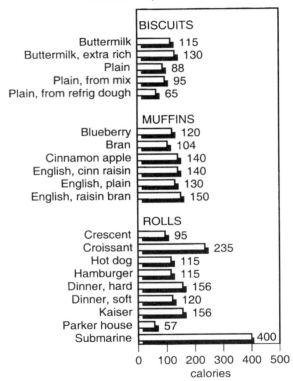

BISCUITS
Buttermilk	115
Buttermilk, extra rich	130
Plain	88
Plain, from mix	95
Plain, from refrig dough	65

MUFFINS
Blueberry	120
Bran	104
Cinnamon apple	140
English, cinn raisin	140
English, plain	130
English, raisin bran	150

ROLLS
Crescent	95
Croissant	235
Hot dog	115
Hamburger	115
Dinner, hard	156
Dinner, soft	120
Kaiser	156
Parker house	57
Submarine	400

0   100   200   300   400   500
calories

* Counts are based on single, average-size items. Average
sweet muffin is assumed to be 2 3/4 inches by 2 inches.
Average sweet and English muffin weight is 57 grams.

Bread, Crackers, and Flours:
BREAD*

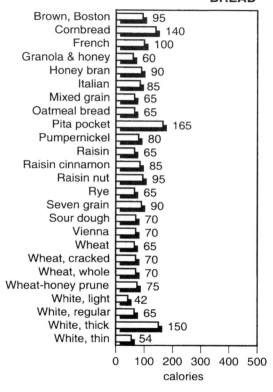

	calories
Brown, Boston	95
Cornbread	140
French	100
Granola & honey	60
Honey bran	90
Italian	85
Mixed grain	65
Oatmeal bread	65
Pita pocket	165
Pumpernickel	80
Raisin	65
Raisin cinnamon	85
Raisin nut	95
Rye	65
Seven grain	90
Sour dough	70
Vienna	70
Wheat	65
Wheat, cracked	70
Wheat, whole	70
Wheat-honey prune	75
White, light	42
White, regular	65
White, thick	150
White, thin	54

* Counts are based on single, average-size slices.

7

Alphabetical Chart
(for Hi-Low Comparison Charts, see pages 83 - 164)

Bread, Crackers, and Flours:
CRACKERS*

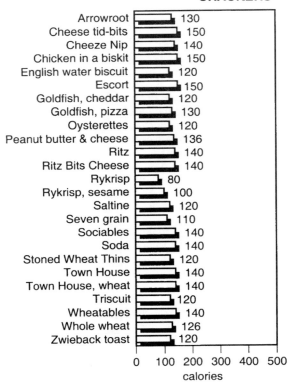

	calories
Arrowroot	130
Cheese tid-bits	150
Cheeze Nip	140
Chicken in a biskit	150
English water biscuit	120
Escort	150
Goldfish, cheddar	120
Goldfish, pizza	130
Oysterettes	120
Peanut butter & cheese	136
Ritz	140
Ritz Bits Cheese	140
Rykrisp	80
Rykrisp, sesame	100
Saltine	120
Seven grain	110
Sociables	140
Soda	140
Stoned Wheat Thins	120
Town House	140
Town House, wheat	140
Triscuit	120
Wheatables	140
Whole wheat	126
Zwieback toast	120

0   100   200   300   400   500
calories

* For ease of comparison, counts are based on one-ounce
servings. Adjust counts to reflect quantities consumed.

Bread, Crackers, and Flours:
DRY & CRISPY*

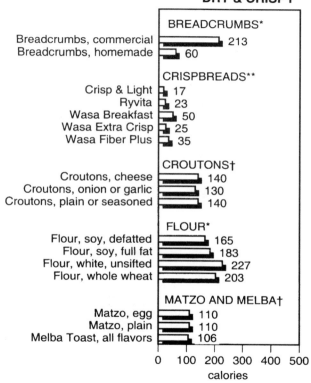

BREADCRUMBS*

Breadcrumbs, commercial	213
Breadcrumbs, homemade	60

CRISPBREADS**

Crisp & Light	17
Ryvita	23
Wasa Breakfast	50
Wasa Extra Crisp	25
Wasa Fiber Plus	35

CROUTONS†

Croutons, cheese	140
Croutons, onion or garlic	130
Croutons, plain or seasoned	140

FLOUR*

Flour, soy, defatted	165
Flour, soy, full fat	183
Flour, white, unsifted	227
Flour, whole wheat	203

MATZO AND MELBA†

Matzo, egg	110
Matzo, plain	110
Melba Toast, all flavors	106

0   100   200   300   400   500
calories

* Counts are based on 1/2- cup servings.
** Counts are based on single item.
† Counts are based on single-ounce servings.

Bread, Crackers, and Flours:
PANCAKES, STUFFING & MORE*

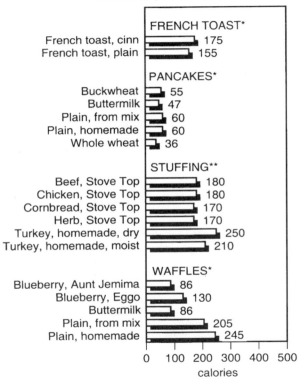

FRENCH TOAST*

French toast, cinn	175
French toast, plain	155

PANCAKES*

Buckwheat	55
Buttermilk	47
Plain, from mix	60
Plain, homemade	60
Whole wheat	36

STUFFING**

Beef, Stove Top	180
Chicken, Stove Top	180
Cornbread, Stove Top	170
Herb, Stove Top	170
Turkey, homemade, dry	250
Turkey, homemade, moist	210

WAFFLES*

Blueberry, Aunt Jemima	86
Blueberry, Eggo	130
Buttermilk	86
Plain, from mix	205
Plain, homemade	245

0   100 200 300 400 500
calories

* Counts are based on a single slice, waffle, or pancake.
** Counts are based on 1/2- cup servings after preparation.

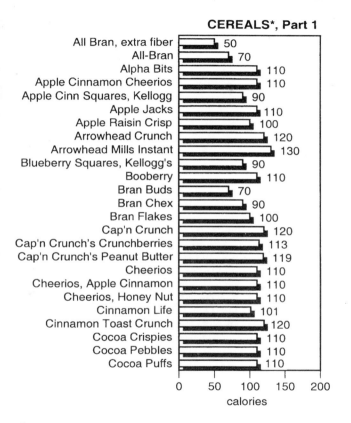

CEREALS*, Part 1

Cereal	calories
All Bran, extra fiber	50
All-Bran	70
Alpha Bits	110
Apple Cinnamon Cheerios	110
Apple Cinn Squares, Kellogg	90
Apple Jacks	110
Apple Raisin Crisp	100
Arrowhead Crunch	120
Arrowhead Mills Instant	130
Blueberry Squares, Kellogg's	90
Booberry	110
Bran Buds	70
Bran Chex	90
Bran Flakes	100
Cap'n Crunch	120
Cap'n Crunch's Crunchberries	113
Cap'n Crunch's Peanut Butter	119
Cheerios	110
Cheerios, Apple Cinnamon	110
Cheerios, Honey Nut	110
Cinnamon Life	101
Cinnamon Toast Crunch	120
Cocoa Crispies	110
Cocoa Pebbles	110
Cocoa Puffs	110

* Counts are based on average-size servings (as indicated on package) and without added milk.

11

CEREALS*, Part 2

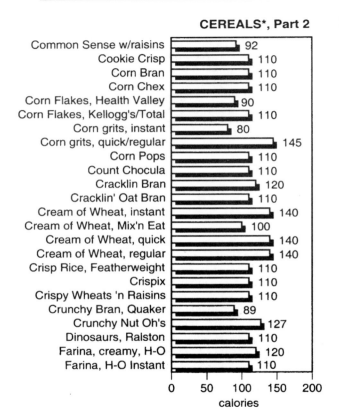

Cereal	calories
Common Sense w/raisins	92
Cookie Crisp	110
Corn Bran	110
Corn Chex	110
Corn Flakes, Health Valley	90
Corn Flakes, Kellogg's/Total	110
Corn grits, instant	80
Corn grits, quick/regular	145
Corn Pops	110
Count Chocula	110
Cracklin Bran	120
Cracklin' Oat Bran	110
Cream of Wheat, instant	140
Cream of Wheat, Mix'n Eat	100
Cream of Wheat, quick	140
Cream of Wheat, regular	140
Crisp Rice, Featherweight	110
Crispix	110
Crispy Wheats 'n Raisins	110
Crunchy Bran, Quaker	89
Crunchy Nut Oh's	127
Dinosaurs, Ralston	110
Farina, creamy, H-O	120
Farina, H-O Instant	110

calories (0 50 100 150 200)

* Counts are based on average-size servings (as indicated on package) and without added milk.

CEREALS*, Part 3

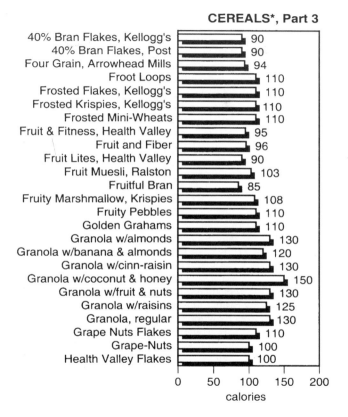

Cereal	calories
40% Bran Flakes, Kellogg's	90
40% Bran Flakes, Post	90
Four Grain, Arrowhead Mills	94
Froot Loops	110
Frosted Flakes, Kellogg's	110
Frosted Krispies, Kellogg's	110
Frosted Mini-Wheats	110
Fruit & Fitness, Health Valley	95
Fruit and Fiber	96
Fruit Lites, Health Valley	90
Fruit Muesli, Ralston	103
Fruitful Bran	85
Fruity Marshmallow, Krispies	108
Fruity Pebbles	110
Golden Grahams	110
Granola w/almonds	130
Granola w/banana & almonds	120
Granola w/cinn-raisin	130
Granola w/coconut & honey	150
Granola w/fruit & nuts	130
Granola w/raisins	125
Granola, regular	130
Grape Nuts Flakes	110
Grape-Nuts	100
Health Valley Flakes	100

calories (0 – 50 – 100 – 150 – 200)

* Counts are based on average-size servings (as indicated
on package) and without added milk.

13

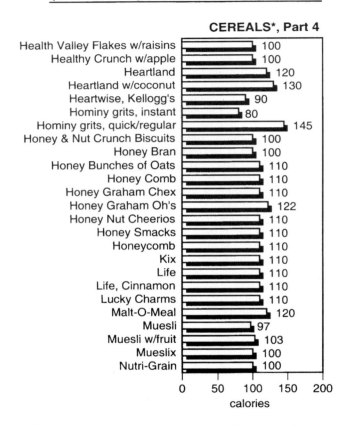

CEREALS*, Part 4

Cereal	calories
Health Valley Flakes w/raisins	100
Healthy Crunch w/apple	100
Heartland	120
Heartland w/coconut	130
Heartwise, Kellogg's	90
Hominy grits, instant	80
Hominy grits, quick/regular	145
Honey & Nut Crunch Biscuits	100
Honey Bran	100
Honey Bunches of Oats	110
Honey Comb	110
Honey Graham Chex	110
Honey Graham Oh's	122
Honey Nut Cheerios	110
Honey Smacks	110
Honeycomb	110
Kix	110
Life	110
Life, Cinnamon	110
Lucky Charms	110
Malt-O-Meal	120
Muesli	97
Muesli w/fruit	103
Mueslix	100
Nutri-Grain	100

* Counts are based on average-size servings (as indicated
on package) and without added milk.

14

CEREALS*, Part 5

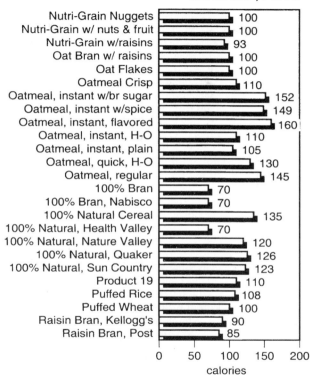

Cereal	calories
Nutri-Grain Nuggets	100
Nutri-Grain w/ nuts & fruit	100
Nutri-Grain w/raisins	93
Oat Bran w/ raisins	100
Oat Flakes	100
Oatmeal Crisp	110
Oatmeal, instant w/br sugar	152
Oatmeal, instant w/spice	149
Oatmeal, instant, flavored	160
Oatmeal, instant, H-O	110
Oatmeal, instant, plain	105
Oatmeal, quick, H-O	130
Oatmeal, regular	145
100% Bran	70
100% Bran, Nabisco	70
100% Natural Cereal	135
100% Natural, Health Valley	70
100% Natural, Nature Valley	120
100% Natural, Quaker	126
100% Natural, Sun Country	123
Product 19	110
Puffed Rice	108
Puffed Wheat	100
Raisin Bran, Kellogg's	90
Raisin Bran, Post	85

* Counts are based on average-size servings (as indicated
  on package) and without added milk.

CEREALS*, Part 6

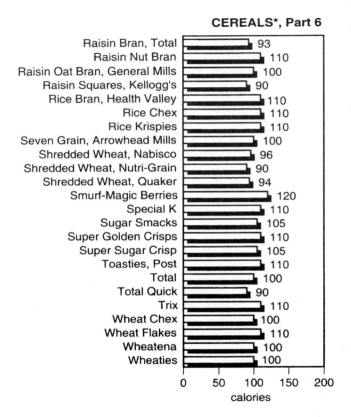

Cereal	calories
Raisin Bran, Total	93
Raisin Nut Bran	110
Raisin Oat Bran, General Mills	100
Raisin Squares, Kellogg's	90
Rice Bran, Health Valley	110
Rice Chex	110
Rice Krispies	110
Seven Grain, Arrowhead Mills	100
Shredded Wheat, Nabisco	96
Shredded Wheat, Nutri-Grain	90
Shredded Wheat, Quaker	94
Smurf-Magic Berries	120
Special K	110
Sugar Smacks	105
Super Golden Crisps	110
Super Sugar Crisp	105
Toasties, Post	110
Total	100
Total Quick	90
Trix	110
Wheat Chex	100
Wheat Flakes	110
Wheatena	100
Wheaties	100

* Counts are based on average-size servings (as indicated
on package) and without added milk.

16

COMBINED AND FROZEN FOODS*, Part 1

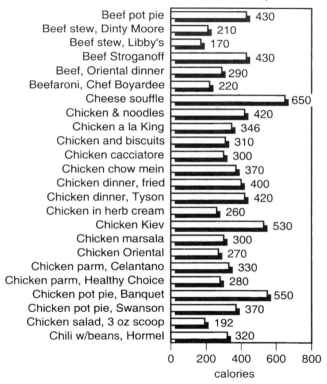

Food	Calories
Beef pot pie	430
Beef stew, Dinty Moore	210
Beef stew, Libby's	170
Beef Stroganoff	430
Beef, Oriental dinner	290
Beefaroni, Chef Boyardee	220
Cheese souffle	650
Chicken & noodles	420
Chicken a la King	346
Chicken and biscuits	310
Chicken cacciatore	300
Chicken chow mein	370
Chicken dinner, fried	400
Chicken dinner, Tyson	420
Chicken in herb cream	260
Chicken Kiev	530
Chicken marsala	300
Chicken Oriental	270
Chicken parm, Celantano	330
Chicken parm, Healthy Choice	280
Chicken pot pie, Banquet	550
Chicken pot pie, Swanson	370
Chicken salad, 3 oz scoop	192
Chili w/beans, Hormel	320

calories

* Counts are based on average-size servings as indicated
on package. Adjust count to reflect amount consumed.

COMBINED AND FROZEN FOODS*,
Part 2

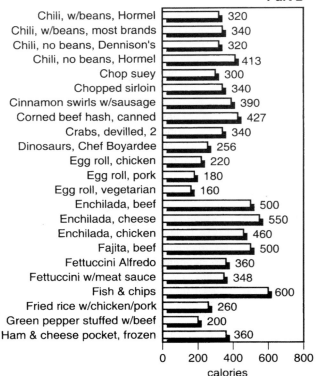

Food	calories
Chili, w/beans, Hormel	320
Chili, w/beans, most brands	340
Chili, no beans, Dennison's	320
Chili, no beans, Hormel	413
Chop suey	300
Chopped sirloin	340
Cinnamon swirls w/sausage	390
Corned beef hash, canned	427
Crabs, devilled, 2	340
Dinosaurs, Chef Boyardee	256
Egg roll, chicken	220
Egg roll, pork	180
Egg roll, vegetarian	160
Enchilada, beef	500
Enchilada, cheese	550
Enchilada, chicken	460
Fajita, beef	500
Fettuccini Alfredo	360
Fettuccini w/meat sauce	348
Fish & chips	600
Fried rice w/chicken/pork	260
Green pepper stuffed w/beef	200
Ham & cheese pocket, frozen	360

calories (0 200 400 600 800)

* Counts are based on average-size servings as indicated
on package. Adjust count to reflect amount consumed.

COMBINED AND FROZEN FOODS*, Part 3

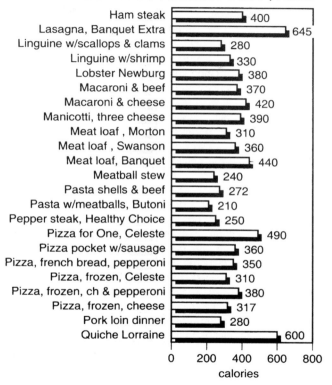

Food	calories
Ham steak	400
Lasagna, Banquet Extra	645
Linguine w/scallops & clams	280
Linguine w/shrimp	330
Lobster Newburg	380
Macaroni & beef	370
Macaroni & cheese	420
Manicotti, three cheese	390
Meat loaf , Morton	310
Meat loaf , Swanson	360
Meat loaf, Banquet	440
Meatball stew	240
Pasta shells & beef	272
Pasta w/meatballs, Butoni	210
Pepper steak, Healthy Choice	250
Pizza for One, Celeste	490
Pizza pocket w/sausage	360
Pizza, french bread, pepperoni	350
Pizza, frozen, Celeste	310
Pizza, frozen, ch & pepperoni	380
Pizza, frozen, cheese	317
Pork loin dinner	280
Quiche Lorraine	600

* Counts are based on average-size servings as indicated
on package. Adjust count to reflect amount consumed.

COMBINED AND FROZEN FOODS*, Part 4

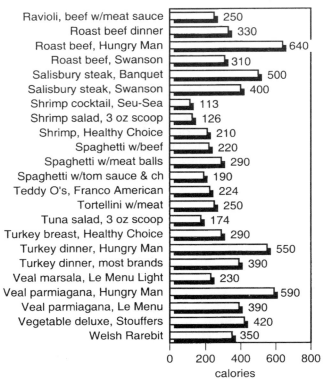

Food	Calories
Ravioli, beef w/meat sauce	250
Roast beef dinner	330
Roast beef, Hungry Man	640
Roast beef, Swanson	310
Salisbury steak, Banquet	500
Salisbury steak, Swanson	400
Shrimp cocktail, Seu-Sea	113
Shrimp salad, 3 oz scoop	126
Shrimp, Healthy Choice	210
Spaghetti w/beef	220
Spaghetti w/meat balls	290
Spaghetti w/tom sauce & ch	190
Teddy O's, Franco American	224
Tortellini w/meat	250
Tuna salad, 3 oz scoop	174
Turkey breast, Healthy Choice	290
Turkey dinner, Hungry Man	550
Turkey dinner, most brands	390
Veal marsala, Le Menu Light	230
Veal parmiagana, Hungry Man	590
Veal parmiagana, Le Menu	390
Vegetable deluxe, Stouffers	420
Welsh Rarebit	350

calories

* Counts are based on average-size servings as indicated
on package. Adjust count to reflect amount consumed.

Dairy: CHEESE (HARD & SEMI-SOFT)*

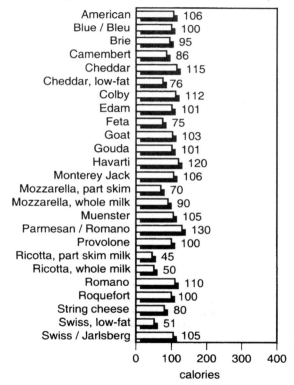

Cheese	calories
American	106
Blue / Bleu	100
Brie	95
Camembert	86
Cheddar	115
Cheddar, low-fat	76
Colby	112
Edam	101
Feta	75
Goat	103
Gouda	101
Havarti	120
Monterey Jack	106
Mozzarella, part skim	70
Mozzarella, whole milk	90
Muenster	105
Parmesan / Romano	130
Provolone	100
Ricotta, part skim milk	45
Ricotta, whole milk	50
Romano	110
Roquefort	100
String cheese	80
Swiss, low-fat	51
Swiss / Jarlsberg	105

calories

* Counts are based on one-ounce servings. Adjust count to
reflect amount consumed.

Dairy: CHEESES (SOFT),, CREAMS & SUBSTITUTES*

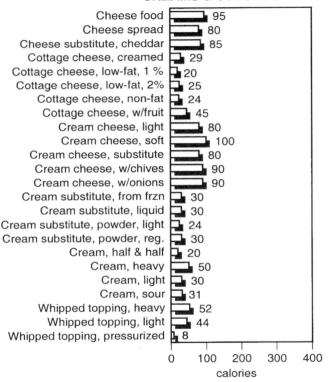

	calories
Cheese food	95
Cheese spread	80
Cheese substitute, cheddar	85
Cottage cheese, creamed	29
Cottage cheese, low-fat, 1 %	20
Cottage cheese, low-fat, 2%	25
Cottage cheese, non-fat	24
Cottage cheese, w/fruit	45
Cream cheese, light	80
Cream cheese, soft	100
Cream cheese, substitute	80
Cream cheese, w/chives	90
Cream cheese, w/onions	90
Cream substitute, from frzn	30
Cream substitute, liquid	30
Cream substitute, powder, light	24
Cream substitute, powder, reg.	30
Cream, half & half	20
Cream, heavy	50
Cream, light	30
Cream, sour	31
Whipped topping, heavy	52
Whipped topping, light	44
Whipped topping, pressurized	8

* Counts are based on one-ounce servings of soft cheese
or one tablespoon of cream or whipped topping.

Dairy: EGGS, MILK, YOGURT & SHAKES*

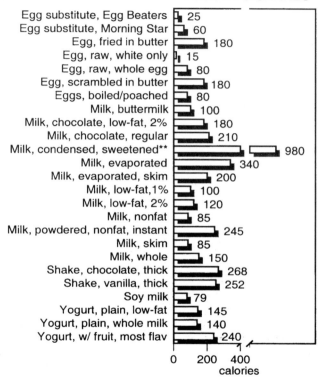

	calories
Egg substitute, Egg Beaters	25
Egg substitute, Morning Star	60
Egg, fried in butter	180
Egg, raw, white only	15
Egg, raw, whole egg	80
Egg, scrambled in butter	180
Eggs, boiled/poached	80
Milk, buttermilk	100
Milk, chocolate, low-fat, 2%	180
Milk, chocolate, regular	210
Milk, condensed, sweetened**	980
Milk, evaporated	340
Milk, evaporated, skim	200
Milk, low-fat,1%	100
Milk, low-fat, 2%	120
Milk, nonfat	85
Milk, powdered, nonfat, instant	245
Milk, skim	85
Milk, whole	150
Shake, chocolate, thick	268
Shake, vanilla, thick	252
Soy milk	79
Yogurt, plain, low-fat	145
Yogurt, plain, whole milk	140
Yogurt, w/ fruit, most flav	240

0   200   400
calories

* Counts are based on one egg or equivalent egg substitute or 8 fluid ounces of milk, yogurt, or shake.
** High count for this item requires break in bar.

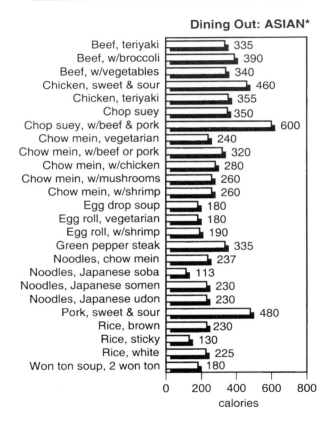

Dining Out: ASIAN*

Item	calories
Beef, teriyaki	335
Beef, w/broccoli	390
Beef, w/vegetables	340
Chicken, sweet & sour	460
Chicken, teriyaki	355
Chop suey	350
Chop suey, w/beef & pork	600
Chow mein, vegetarian	240
Chow mein, w/beef or pork	320
Chow mein, w/chicken	280
Chow mein, w/mushrooms	260
Chow mein, w/shrimp	260
Egg drop soup	180
Egg roll, vegetarian	180
Egg roll, w/shrimp	190
Green pepper steak	335
Noodles, chow mein	237
Noodles, Japanese soba	113
Noodles, Japanese somen	230
Noodles, Japanese udon	230
Pork, sweet & sour	480
Rice, brown	230
Rice, sticky	130
Rice, white	225
Won ton soup, 2 won ton	180

* Counts based on average-sized servings (for main dishes,
1 1/2 - 2 cups). Counts for main dishes include rice.

Dining Out: DELICATESSEN*

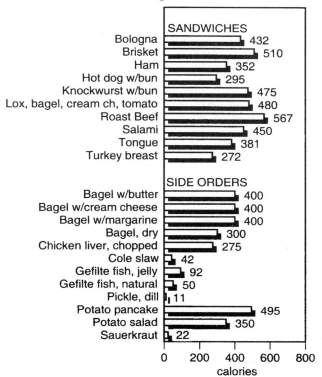

SANDWICHES

	calories
Bologna	432
Brisket	510
Ham	352
Hot dog w/bun	295
Knockwurst w/bun	475
Lox, bagel, cream ch, tomato	480
Roast Beef	567
Salami	450
Tongue	381
Turkey breast	272

SIDE ORDERS

	calories
Bagel w/butter	400
Bagel w/cream cheese	400
Bagel w/margarine	400
Bagel, dry	300
Chicken liver, chopped	275
Cole slaw	42
Gefilte fish, jelly	92
Gefilte fish, natural	50
Pickle, dill	11
Potato pancake	495
Potato salad	350
Sauerkraut	22

0   200   400   600   800
calories

* Unless otherwise indicated, counts based on average-
  size servings or sandwiches. Sandwich counts assume
  white or rye bread.

Dining Out: FRENCH AND OTHER INTERNATIONAL DISHES*

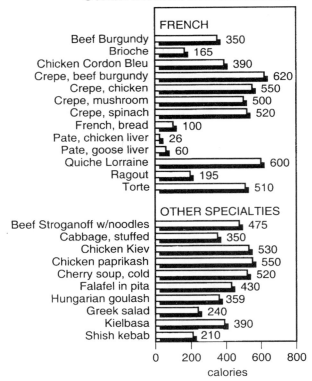

FRENCH

Dish	Calories
Beef Burgundy	350
Brioche	165
Chicken Cordon Bleu	390
Crepe, beef burgundy	620
Crepe, chicken	550
Crepe, mushroom	500
Crepe, spinach	520
French, bread	100
Pate, chicken liver	26
Pate, goose liver	60
Quiche Lorraine	600
Ragout	195
Torte	510

OTHER SPECIALTIES

Dish	Calories
Beef Stroganoff w/noodles	475
Cabbage, stuffed	350
Chicken Kiev	530
Chicken paprikash	550
Cherry soup, cold	520
Falafel in pita	430
Hungarian goulash	359
Greek salad	240
Kielbasa	390
Shish kebab	210

calories: 0   200   400   600   800

* Counts based on average-sized servings (for main dishes, 1 1/2 - 2 cups).

Dining Out: ITALIAN*

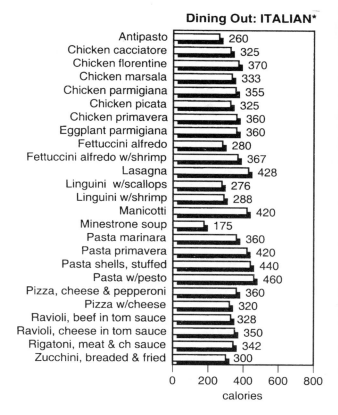

Item	calories
Antipasto	260
Chicken cacciatore	325
Chicken florentine	370
Chicken marsala	333
Chicken parmigiana	355
Chicken picata	325
Chicken primavera	360
Eggplant parmigiana	360
Fettuccini alfredo	280
Fettuccini alfredo w/shrimp	367
Lasagna	428
Linguini w/scallops	276
Linguini w/shrimp	288
Manicotti	420
Minestrone soup	175
Pasta marinara	360
Pasta primavera	420
Pasta shells, stuffed	440
Pasta w/pesto	460
Pizza, cheese & pepperoni	360
Pizza w/cheese	320
Ravioli, beef in tom sauce	328
Ravioli, cheese in tom sauce	350
Rigatoni, meat & ch sauce	342
Zucchini, breaded & fried	300

* Counts are based on average-sized servings (1 1/2 - 2
cups); for pizza, on 1/6 medium or 1/8 large pizza).

Dining Out: MEXICAN*

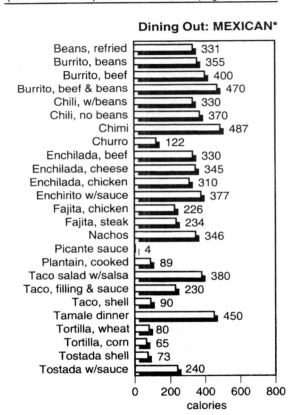

Food	calories
Beans, refried	331
Burrito, beans	355
Burrito, beef	400
Burrito, beef & beans	470
Chili, w/beans	330
Chili, no beans	370
Chimi	487
Churro	122
Enchilada, beef	330
Enchilada, cheese	345
Enchilada, chicken	310
Enchirito w/sauce	377
Fajita, chicken	226
Fajita, steak	234
Nachos	346
Picante sauce	4
Plantain, cooked	89
Taco salad w/salsa	380
Taco, filling & sauce	230
Taco, shell	90
Tamale dinner	450
Tortilla, wheat	80
Tortilla, corn	65
Tostada shell	73
Tostada w/sauce	240

* Counts based on average-sized servings (for main dishes,
1 1/2 - 2 cups).

Fast Food: ARBY'S*

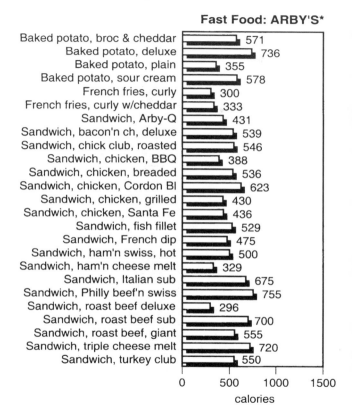

Item	calories
Baked potato, broc & cheddar	571
Baked potato, deluxe	736
Baked potato, plain	355
Baked potato, sour cream	578
French fries, curly	300
French fries, curly w/cheddar	333
Sandwich, Arby-Q	431
Sandwich, bacon'n ch, deluxe	539
Sandwich, chick club, roasted	546
Sandwich, chicken, BBQ	388
Sandwich, chicken, breaded	536
Sandwich, chicken, Cordon Bl	623
Sandwich, chicken, grilled	430
Sandwich, chicken, Santa Fe	436
Sandwich, fish fillet	529
Sandwich, French dip	475
Sandwich, ham'n swiss, hot	500
Sandwich, ham'n cheese melt	329
Sandwich, Italian sub	675
Sandwich, Philly beef'n swiss	755
Sandwich, roast beef deluxe	296
Sandwich, roast beef sub	700
Sandwich, roast beef, giant	555
Sandwich, triple cheese melt	720
Sandwich, turkey club	550

* Unless otherwise indicated, counts are based on average-size servings.

Alphabetical Chart
(for Hi-Low Comparison Charts, see pages 83 - 164)

Fast Food: BOSTON MARKET*

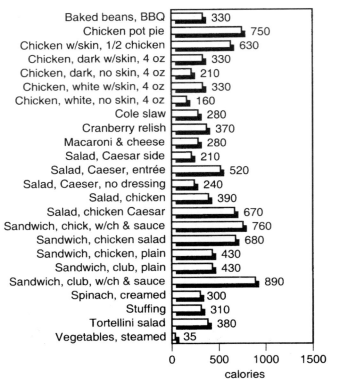

	calories
Baked beans, BBQ	330
Chicken pot pie	750
Chicken w/skin, 1/2 chicken	630
Chicken, dark w/skin, 4 oz	330
Chicken, dark, no skin, 4 oz	210
Chicken, white w/skin, 4 oz	330
Chicken, white, no skin, 4 oz	160
Cole slaw	280
Cranberry relish	370
Macaroni & cheese	280
Salad, Caesar side	210
Salad, Caeser, entrée	520
Salad, Caeser, no dressing	240
Salad, chicken	390
Salad, chicken Caesar	670
Sandwich, chick, w/ch & sauce	760
Sandwich, chicken salad	680
Sandwich, chicken, plain	430
Sandwich, club, plain	430
Sandwich, club, w/ch & sauce	890
Spinach, creamed	300
Stuffing	310
Tortellini salad	380
Vegetables, steamed	35

* Unless otherwise indicated, counts are based on average-size servings.

30

Fast Food: BURGER KING*

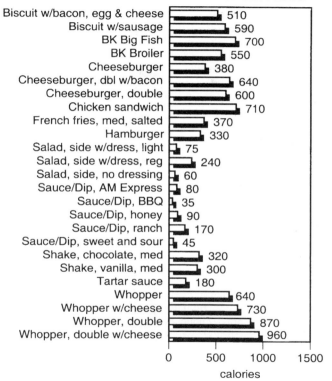

Item	calories
Biscuit w/bacon, egg & cheese	510
Biscuit w/sausage	590
BK Big Fish	700
BK Broiler	550
Cheeseburger	380
Cheeseburger, dbl w/bacon	640
Cheeseburger, double	600
Chicken sandwich	710
French fries, med, salted	370
Hamburger	330
Salad, side w/dress, light	75
Salad, side w/dress, reg	240
Salad, side, no dressing	60
Sauce/Dip, AM Express	80
Sauce/Dip, BBQ	35
Sauce/Dip, honey	90
Sauce/Dip, ranch	170
Sauce/Dip, sweet and sour	45
Shake, chocolate, med	320
Shake, vanilla, med	300
Tartar sauce	180
Whopper	640
Whopper w/cheese	730
Whopper, double	870
Whopper, double w/cheese	960

* Unless otherwise indicated, counts are based on average-size servings.

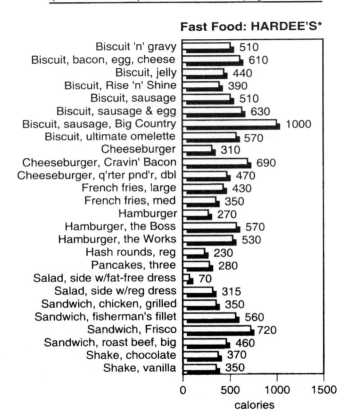

Alphabetical Chart
(for Hi-Low Comparison Charts, see pages 83 - 164)

Fast Food: HARDEE'S*

Item	Calories
Biscuit 'n' gravy	510
Biscuit, bacon, egg, cheese	610
Biscuit, jelly	440
Biscuit, Rise 'n' Shine	390
Biscuit, sausage	510
Biscuit, sausage & egg	630
Biscuit, sausage, Big Country	1000
Biscuit, ultimate omelette	570
Cheeseburger	310
Cheeseburger, Cravin' Bacon	690
Cheeseburger, q'rter pnd'r, dbl	470
French fries, large	430
French fries, med	350
Hamburger	270
Hamburger, the Boss	570
Hamburger, the Works	530
Hash rounds, reg	230
Pancakes, three	280
Salad, side w/fat-free dress	70
Salad, side w/reg dress	315
Sandwich, chicken, grilled	350
Sandwich, fisherman's fillet	560
Sandwich, Frisco	720
Sandwich, roast beef, big	460
Shake, chocolate	370
Shake, vanilla	350

calories

* Unless otherwise indicated, counts are based on average-size servings.

32

Fast Food: JACK IN THE BOX*

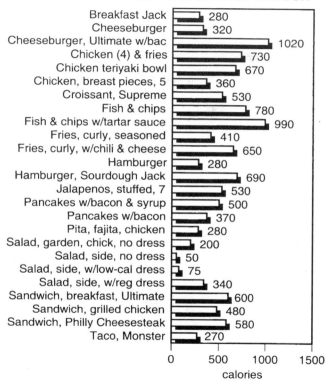

Item	calories
Breakfast Jack	280
Cheeseburger	320
Cheeseburger, Ultimate w/bac	1020
Chicken (4) & fries	730
Chicken teriyaki bowl	670
Chicken, breast pieces, 5	360
Croissant, Supreme	530
Fish & chips	780
Fish & chips w/tartar sauce	990
Fries, curly, seasoned	410
Fries, curly, w/chili & cheese	650
Hamburger	280
Hamburger, Sourdough Jack	690
Jalapenos, stuffed, 7	530
Pancakes w/bacon & syrup	500
Pancakes w/bacon	370
Pita, fajita, chicken	280
Salad, garden, chick, no dress	200
Salad, side, no dress	50
Salad, side, w/low-cal dress	75
Salad, side, w/reg dress	340
Sandwich, breakfast, Ultimate	600
Sandwich, grilled chicken	480
Sandwich, Philly Cheesesteak	580
Taco, Monster	270

calories

* Unless otherwise indicated, counts are based on average-
size servings.

Fast Food: KFC*

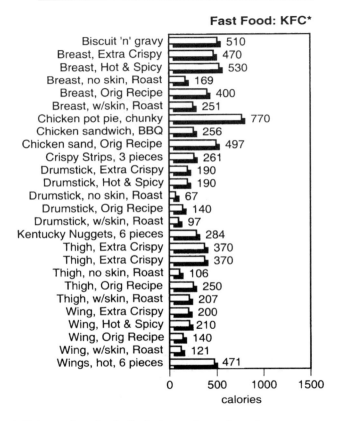

	calories
Biscuit 'n' gravy	510
Breast, Extra Crispy	470
Breast, Hot & Spicy	530
Breast, no skin, Roast	169
Breast, Orig Recipe	400
Breast, w/skin, Roast	251
Chicken pot pie, chunky	770
Chicken sandwich, BBQ	256
Chicken sand, Orig Recipe	497
Crispy Strips, 3 pieces	261
Drumstick, Extra Crispy	190
Drumstick, Hot & Spicy	190
Drumstick, no skin, Roast	67
Drumstick, Orig Recipe	140
Drumstick, w/skin, Roast	97
Kentucky Nuggets, 6 pieces	284
Thigh, Extra Crispy	370
Thigh, Extra Crispy	370
Thigh, no skin, Roast	106
Thigh, Orig Recipe	250
Thigh, w/skin, Roast	207
Wing, Extra Crispy	200
Wing, Hot & Spicy	210
Wing, Orig Recipe	140
Wing, w/skin, Roast	121
Wings, hot, 6 pieces	471

* Unless otherwise indicated, counts are based on average-
size servings.

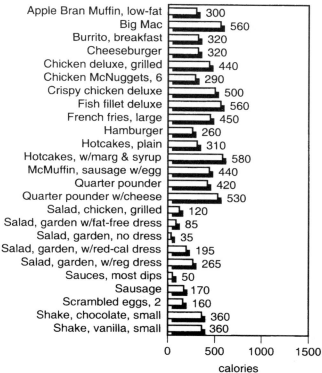

Fast Food: MC DONALD'S*

Item	Calories
Apple Bran Muffin, low-fat	300
Big Mac	560
Burrito, breakfast	320
Cheeseburger	320
Chicken deluxe, grilled	440
Chicken McNuggets, 6	290
Crispy chicken deluxe	500
Fish fillet deluxe	560
French fries, large	450
Hamburger	260
Hotcakes, plain	310
Hotcakes, w/marg & syrup	580
McMuffin, sausage w/egg	440
Quarter pounder	420
Quarter pounder w/cheese	530
Salad, chicken, grilled	120
Salad, garden w/fat-free dress	85
Salad, garden, no dress	35
Salad, garden, w/red-cal dress	195
Salad, garden, w/reg dress	265
Sauces, most dips	50
Sausage	170
Scrambled eggs, 2	160
Shake, chocolate, small	360
Shake, vanilla, small	360

0   500   1000   1500

calories

* Unless otherwise indicated, counts are based on average-
size servings.

Alphabetical Chart
(for Hi-Low Comparison Charts, see pages 83 - 164)

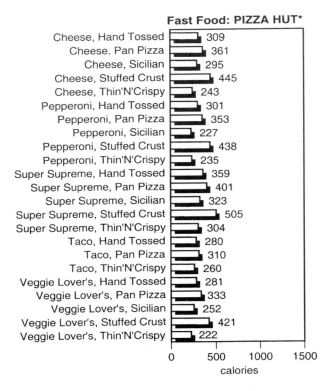

Fast Food: PIZZA HUT*

	calories
Cheese, Hand Tossed	309
Cheese, Pan Pizza	361
Cheese, Sicilian	295
Cheese, Stuffed Crust	445
Cheese, Thin'N'Crispy	243
Pepperoni, Hand Tossed	301
Pepperoni, Pan Pizza	353
Pepperoni, Sicilian	227
Pepperoni, Stuffed Crust	438
Pepperoni, Thin'N'Crispy	235
Super Supreme, Hand Tossed	359
Super Supreme, Pan Pizza	401
Super Supreme, Sicilian	323
Super Supreme, Stuffed Crust	505
Super Supreme, Thin'N'Crispy	304
Taco, Hand Tossed	280
Taco, Pan Pizza	310
Taco, Thin'N'Crispy	260
Veggie Lover's, Hand Tossed	281
Veggie Lover's, Pan Pizza	333
Veggie Lover's, Sicilian	252
Veggie Lover's, Stuffed Crust	421
Veggie Lover's, Thin'N'Crispy	222

* Unless otherwise indicated, counts are based on average-size servings.

Fast Food: SUBWAY*

	calories
Chicken taco subway, wheat	436
Chicken taco subway, white	421
Club, wheat	312
Club, white	297
Cold Cut Trio, wheat	378
Cold Cut Trio, white	362
Meatball, wheat	419
Meatball, white	404
Pizza Sub, wheat	464
Pizza Sub, white	448
Roast beef, wheat	303
Roast beef, white	288
Seafood & crab, wheat	430
Seafood & crab, white	415
Spicy Italian, wheat	482
Spicy Italian, white	467
Steak & cheese, wheat	398
Steak & cheese, white	383
Tuna, wheat	542
Tuna, white	527
Turkey, wheat	289
Turkey, white	273
Veggie Delite, wheat	237
Veggie Delite, white	222

0   500   1000   1500
calories

* Unless otherwise indicated, counts are based on average-
  size servings.

37

Fast Food: TACO BELL*

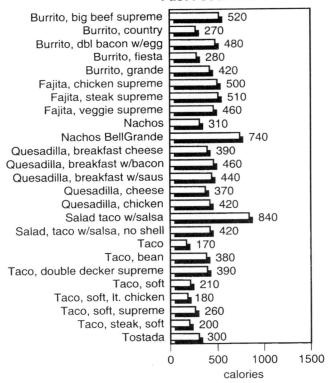

Item	Calories
Burrito, big beef supreme	520
Burrito, country	270
Burrito, dbl bacon w/egg	480
Burrito, fiesta	280
Burrito, grande	420
Fajita, chicken supreme	500
Fajita, steak supreme	510
Fajita, veggie supreme	460
Nachos	310
Nachos BellGrande	740
Quesadilla, breakfast cheese	390
Quesadilla, breakfast w/bacon	460
Quesadilla, breakfast w/saus	440
Quesadilla, cheese	370
Quesadilla, chicken	420
Salad taco w/salsa	840
Salad, taco w/salsa, no shell	420
Taco	170
Taco, bean	380
Taco, double decker supreme	390
Taco, soft	210
Taco, soft, lt. chicken	180
Taco, soft, supreme	260
Taco, steak, soft	200
Tostada	300

calories

* Unless otherwise indicated, counts are based on average-size servings.

Fast Food: WENDY'S*

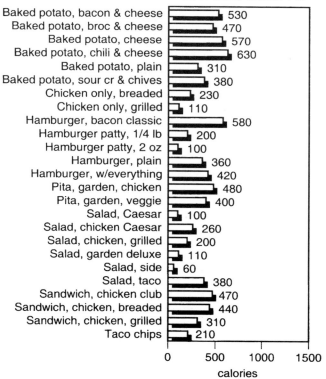

Item	calories
Baked potato, bacon & cheese	530
Baked potato, broc & cheese	470
Baked potato, cheese	570
Baked potato, chili & cheese	630
Baked potato, plain	310
Baked potato, sour cr & chives	380
Chicken only, breaded	230
Chicken only, grilled	110
Hamburger, bacon classic	580
Hamburger patty, 1/4 lb	200
Hamburger patty, 2 oz	100
Hamburger, plain	360
Hamburger, w/everything	420
Pita, garden, chicken	480
Pita, garden, veggie	400
Salad, Caesar	100
Salad, chicken Caesar	260
Salad, chicken, grilled	200
Salad, garden deluxe	110
Salad, side	60
Salad, taco	380
Sandwich, chicken club	470
Sandwich, chicken, breaded	440
Sandwich, chicken, grilled	310
Taco chips	210

calories (0, 500, 1000, 1500)

* Unless otherwise indicated, counts are based on average-
size servings.

Fruits: FRESH & DRIED FRUITS AND JUICES *, Part 1

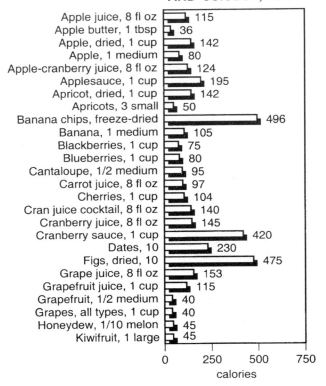

Food	calories
Apple juice, 8 fl oz	115
Apple butter, 1 tbsp	36
Apple, dried, 1 cup	142
Apple, 1 medium	80
Apple-cranberry juice, 8 fl oz	124
Applesauce, 1 cup	195
Apricot, dried, 1 cup	142
Apricots, 3 small	50
Banana chips, freeze-dried	496
Banana, 1 medium	105
Blackberries, 1 cup	75
Blueberries, 1 cup	80
Cantaloupe, 1/2 medium	95
Carrot juice, 8 fl oz	97
Cherries, 1 cup	104
Cran juice cocktail, 8 fl oz	140
Cranberry juice, 8 fl oz	145
Cranberry sauce, 1 cup	420
Dates, 10	230
Figs, dried, 10	475
Grape juice, 8 fl oz	153
Grapefruit juice, 1 cup	115
Grapefruit, 1/2 medium	40
Grapes, all types, 1 cup	40
Honeydew, 1/10 melon	45
Kiwifruit, 1 large	45

calories (0, 250, 500, 750)

* Unless otherwise indicated, counts are based on whole, fresh fruits.

40

Fruits: FRESH & DRIED FRUITS
AND JUICES *, Part 2

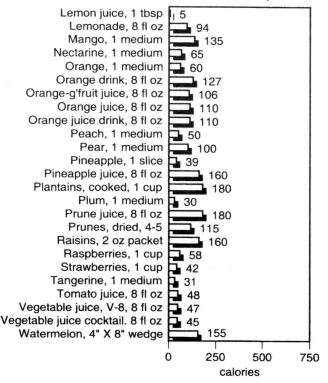

Food	calories
Lemon juice, 1 tbsp	5
Lemonade, 8 fl oz	94
Mango, 1 medium	135
Nectarine, 1 medium	65
Orange, 1 medium	60
Orange drink, 8 fl oz	127
Orange-g'fruit juice, 8 fl oz	106
Orange juice, 8 fl oz	110
Orange juice drink, 8 fl oz	110
Peach, 1 medium	50
Pear, 1 medium	100
Pineapple, 1 slice	39
Pineapple juice, 8 fl oz	160
Plantains, cooked, 1 cup	180
Plum, 1 medium	30
Prune juice, 8 fl oz	180
Prunes, dried, 4-5	115
Raisins, 2 oz packet	160
Raspberries, 1 cup	58
Strawberries, 1 cup	42
Tangerine, 1 medium	31
Tomato juice, 8 fl oz	48
Vegetable juice, V-8, 8 fl oz	47
Vegetable juice cocktail. 8 fl oz	45
Watermelon, 4" X 8" wedge	155

calories (0 – 250 – 500 – 750)

* Unless otherwise indicated, counts are based on whole, fresh fruits.

41

GRAVIES, SAUCES & DIPS*

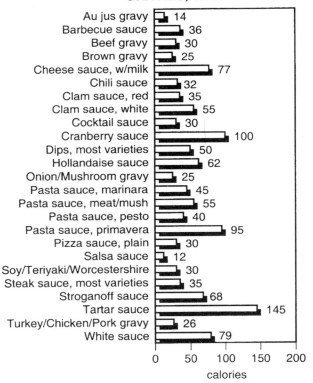

	calories
Au jus gravy	14
Barbecue sauce	36
Beef gravy	30
Brown gravy	25
Cheese sauce, w/milk	77
Chili sauce	32
Clam sauce, red	35
Clam sauce, white	55
Cocktail sauce	30
Cranberry sauce	100
Dips, most varieties	50
Hollandaise sauce	62
Onion/Mushroom gravy	25
Pasta sauce, marinara	45
Pasta sauce, meat/mush	55
Pasta sauce, pesto	40
Pasta sauce, primavera	95
Pizza sauce, plain	30
Salsa sauce	12
Soy/Teriyaki/Worcestershire	30
Steak sauce, most varieties	35
Stroganoff sauce	68
Tartar sauce	145
Turkey/Chicken/Pork gravy	26
White sauce	79

*Counts are based on one-quarter cup servings.

MEATS*, Part 1

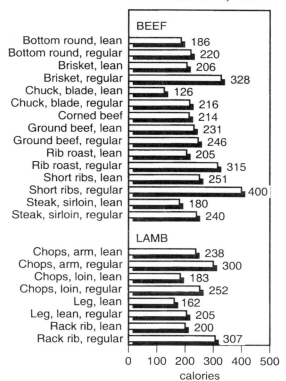

BEEF

	calories
Bottom round, lean	186
Bottom round, regular	220
Brisket, lean	206
Brisket, regular	328
Chuck, blade, lean	126
Chuck, blade, regular	216
Corned beef	214
Ground beef, lean	231
Ground beef, regular	246
Rib roast, lean	205
Rib roast, regular	315
Short ribs, lean	251
Short ribs, regular	400
Steak, sirloin, lean	180
Steak, sirloin, regular	240

LAMB

	calories
Chops, arm, lean	238
Chops, arm, regular	300
Chops, loin, lean	183
Chops, loin, regular	252
Leg, lean	162
Leg, lean, regular	205
Rack rib, lean	200
Rack rib, regular	307

0   100   200   300   400   500
calories

* Counts are based on 3-ounce servings.

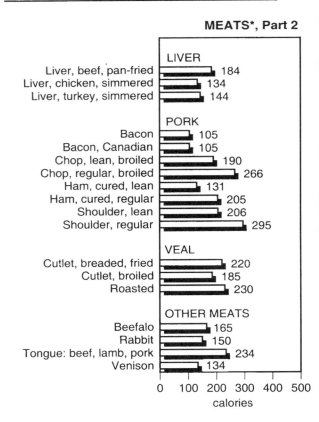

MEATS*, Part 2

LIVER

Liver, beef, pan-fried	184
Liver, chicken, simmered	134
Liver, turkey, simmered	144

PORK

Bacon	105
Bacon, Canadian	105
Chop, lean, broiled	190
Chop, regular, broiled	266
Ham, cured, lean	131
Ham, cured, regular	205
Shoulder, lean	206
Shoulder, regular	295

VEAL

Cutlet, breaded, fried	220
Cutlet, broiled	185
Roasted	230

OTHER MEATS

Beefalo	165
Rabbit	150
Tongue: beef, lamb, pork	234
Venison	134

0   100   200   300   400   500
calories

* Counts are based on 3-ounce servings.

44

MEATS, PROCESSED*

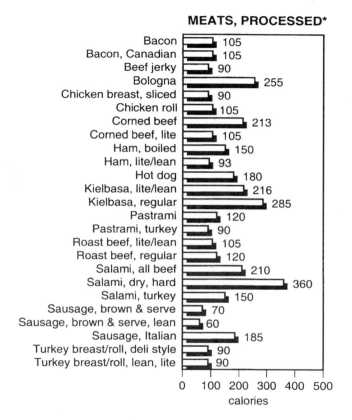

Food	calories
Bacon	105
Bacon, Canadian	105
Beef jerky	90
Bologna	255
Chicken breast, sliced	90
Chicken roll	105
Corned beef	213
Corned beef, lite	105
Ham, boiled	150
Ham, lite/lean	93
Hot dog	180
Kielbasa, lite/lean	216
Kielbasa, regular	285
Pastrami	120
Pastrami, turkey	90
Roast beef, lite/lean	105
Roast beef, regular	120
Salami, all beef	210
Salami, dry, hard	360
Salami, turkey	150
Sausage, brown & serve	70
Sausage, brown & serve, lean	60
Sausage, Italian	185
Turkey breast/roll, deli style	90
Turkey breast/roll, lean, lite	90

* Counts are based on 3-ounce servings.

45

Medications: COUGH DROPS & SYRUPS*

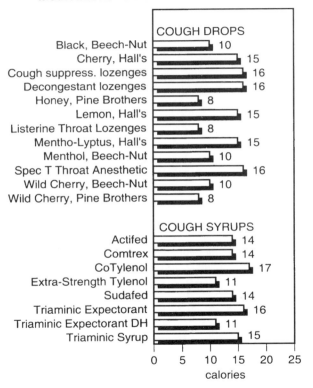

COUGH DROPS

	calories
Black, Beech-Nut	10
Cherry, Hall's	15
Cough suppress. lozenges	16
Decongestant lozenges	16
Honey, Pine Brothers	8
Lemon, Hall's	15
Listerine Throat Lozenges	8
Mentho-Lyptus, Hall's	15
Menthol, Beech-Nut	10
Spec T Throat Anesthetic	16
Wild Cherry, Beech-Nut	10
Wild Cherry, Pine Brothers	8

COUGH SYRUPS

	calories
Actifed	14
Comtrex	14
CoTylenol	17
Extra-Strength Tylenol	11
Sudafed	14
Triaminic Expectorant	16
Triaminic Expectorant DH	11
Triaminic Syrup	15

calories

* Counts are based on one cough drops or on recommended
doses for adults.

Medications: OVER-THE-COUNTER REMEDIES & VITAMINS AND MINERALS*

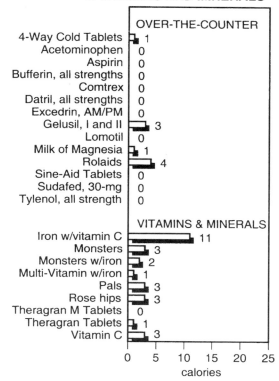

OVER-THE-COUNTER

4-Way Cold Tablets	1
Acetominophen	0
Aspirin	0
Bufferin, all strengths	0
Comtrex	0
Datril, all strengths	0
Excedrin, AM/PM	0
Gelusil, I and II	3
Lomotil	0
Milk of Magnesia	1
Rolaids	4
Sine-Aid Tablets	0
Sudafed, 30-mg	0
Tylenol, all strength	0

VITAMINS & MINERALS

Iron w/vitamin C	11
Monsters	3
Monsters w/iron	2
Multi-Vitamin w/iron	1
Pals	3
Rose hips	3
Theragran M Tablets	0
Theragran Tablets	1
Vitamin C	3

0   5   10   15   20   25
calories

* Counts are based on recommended doses for adults.

Alphabetical Chart
(for Hi-Low Comparison Charts, see pages 83 - 164)

MISCELLANEOUS FOODS*

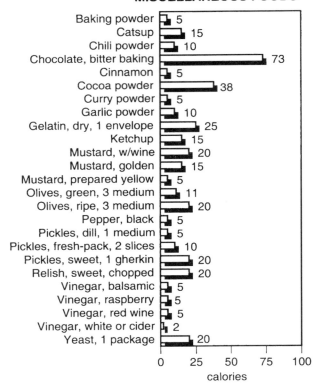

Food	calories
Baking powder	5
Catsup	15
Chili powder	10
Chocolate, bitter baking	73
Cinnamon	5
Cocoa powder	38
Curry powder	5
Garlic powder	10
Gelatin, dry, 1 envelope	25
Ketchup	15
Mustard, w/wine	20
Mustard, golden	15
Mustard, prepared yellow	5
Olives, green, 3 medium	11
Olives, ripe, 3 medium	20
Pepper, black	5
Pickles, dill, 1 medium	5
Pickles, fresh-pack, 2 slices	10
Pickles, sweet, 1 gherkin	20
Relish, sweet, chopped	20
Vinegar, balsamic	5
Vinegar, raspberry	5
Vinegar, red wine	5
Vinegar, white or cider	2
Yeast, 1 package	20

* Unless otherwise indicated, counts are based on
  a one-tablespoon serving.

NUTS, BEANS AND SEEDS*: Part 1

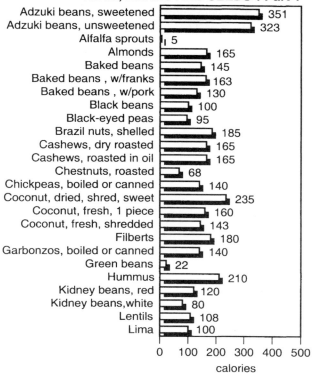

Food	calories
Adzuki beans, sweetened	351
Adzuki beans, unsweetened	323
Alfalfa sprouts	5
Almonds	165
Baked beans	145
Baked beans , w/franks	163
Baked beans , w/pork	130
Black beans	100
Black-eyed peas	95
Brazil nuts, shelled	185
Cashews, dry roasted	165
Cashews, roasted in oil	165
Chestnuts, roasted	68
Chickpeas, boiled or canned	140
Coconut, dried, shred, sweet	235
Coconut, fresh, 1 piece	160
Coconut, fresh, shredded	143
Filberts	180
Garbonzos, boiled or canned	140
Green beans	22
Hummus	210
Kidney beans, red	120
Kidney beans,white	80
Lentils	108
Lima	100

calories (0 100 200 300 400 500)

* Unless otherwise indicated, counts are based on 1/2 cup
tofu or cooked beans or one-ounce servings of raw nuts or
seeds.

NUTS, BEANS AND SEEDS*: Part 2

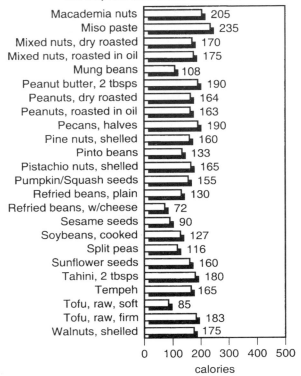

	calories
Macadamia nuts	205
Miso paste	235
Mixed nuts, dry roasted	170
Mixed nuts, roasted in oil	175
Mung beans	108
Peanut butter, 2 tbsps	190
Peanuts, dry roasted	164
Peanuts, roasted in oil	163
Pecans, halves	190
Pine nuts, shelled	160
Pinto beans	133
Pistachio nuts, shelled	165
Pumpkin/Squash seeds	155
Refried beans, plain	130
Refried beans, w/cheese	72
Sesame seeds	90
Soybeans, cooked	127
Split peas	116
Sunflower seeds	160
Tahini, 2 tbsps	180
Tempeh	165
Tofu, raw, soft	85
Tofu, raw, firm	183
Walnuts, shelled	175

0 100 200 300 400 500
calories

* Unless otherwise indicated, counts are based on 1/2 cup
tofu or cooked beans or one-ounce servings of raw nuts or
seeds.

OILS AND FATS*

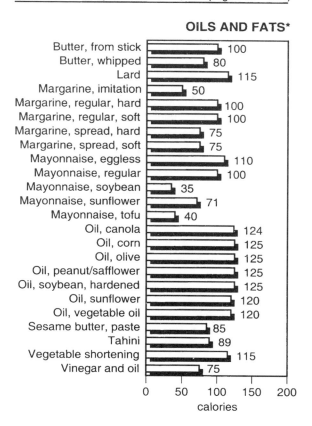

	calories
Butter, from stick	100
Butter, whipped	80
Lard	115
Margarine, imitation	50
Margarine, regular, hard	100
Margarine, regular, soft	100
Margarine, spread, hard	75
Margarine, spread, soft	75
Mayonnaise, eggless	110
Mayonnaise, regular	100
Mayonnaise, soybean	35
Mayonnaise, sunflower	71
Mayonnaise, tofu	40
Oil, canola	124
Oil, corn	125
Oil, olive	125
Oil, peanut/safflower	125
Oil, soybean, hardened	125
Oil, sunflower	120
Oil, vegetable oil	120
Sesame butter, paste	85
Tahini	89
Vegetable shortening	115
Vinegar and oil	75

* Counts are based on 1-tablespoon servings.

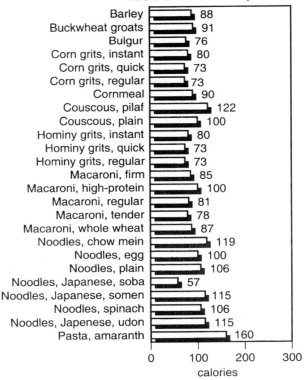

PASTA, WHOLE GRAINS , RICE & NOODLES*, Part 1

	calories
Barley	88
Buckwheat groats	91
Bulgur	76
Corn grits, instant	80
Corn grits, quick	73
Corn grits, regular	73
Cornmeal	90
Couscous, pilaf	122
Couscous, plain	100
Hominy grits, instant	80
Hominy grits, quick	73
Hominy grits, regular	73
Macaroni, firm	85
Macaroni, high-protein	100
Macaroni, regular	81
Macaroni, tender	78
Macaroni, whole wheat	87
Noodles, chow mein	119
Noodles, egg	100
Noodles, plain	106
Noodles, Japanese, soba	57
Noodles, Japanese, somen	115
Noodles, spinach	106
Noodles, Japenese, udon	115
Pasta, amaranth	160

calories (0, 100, 200, 300)

* Counts based on cooked, 1/2-cup servings.

PASTA, WHOLE GRAINS , RICE & NOODLES*, Part 2

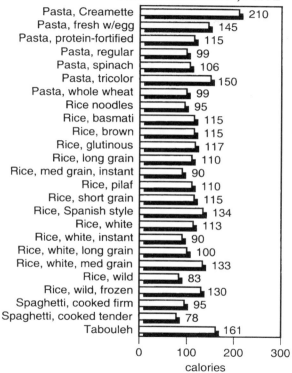

	calories
Pasta, Creamette	210
Pasta, fresh w/egg	145
Pasta, protein-fortified	115
Pasta, regular	99
Pasta, spinach	106
Pasta, tricolor	150
Pasta, whole wheat	99
Rice noodles	95
Rice, basmati	115
Rice, brown	115
Rice, glutinous	117
Rice, long grain	110
Rice, med grain, instant	90
Rice, pilaf	110
Rice, short grain	115
Rice, Spanish style	134
Rice, white	113
Rice, white, instant	90
Rice, white, long grain	100
Rice, white, med grain	133
Rice, wild	83
Rice, wild, frozen	130
Spaghetti, cooked firm	95
Spaghetti, cooked tender	78
Tabouleh	161

* Counts based on cooked, 1/2-cup servings.

Poultry: CHICKEN, TURKEY, AND OTHER FOWL*

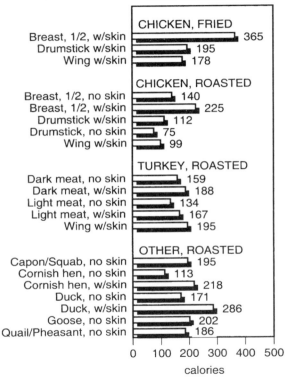

CHICKEN, FRIED

Breast, 1/2, w/skin	365
Drumstick w/skin	195
Wing w/skin	178

CHICKEN, ROASTED

Breast, 1/2, no skin	140
Breast, 1/2, w/skin	225
Drumstick w/skin	112
Drumstick, no skin	75
Wing w/skin	99

TURKEY, ROASTED

Dark meat, no skin	159
Dark meat, w/skin	188
Light meat, no skin	134
Light meat, w/skin	167
Wing w/skin	195

OTHER, ROASTED

Capon/Squab, no skin	195
Cornish hen, no skin	113
Cornish hen, w/skin	218
Duck, no skin	171
Duck, w/skin	286
Goose, no skin	202
Quail/Pheasant, no skin	186

0   100   200   300   400   500

calories

* Unless otherwise indicated, counts are based on 3-ounce servings.

54

SALAD BAR CHOICES*

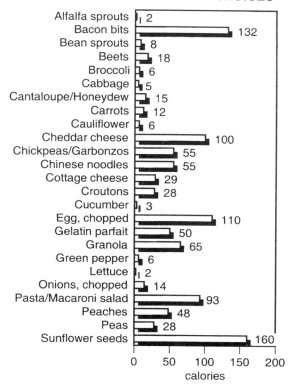

Salad Bar Choice	calories
Alfalfa sprouts	2
Bacon bits	132
Bean sprouts	8
Beets	18
Broccoli	6
Cabbage	5
Cantaloupe/Honeydew	15
Carrots	12
Cauliflower	6
Cheddar cheese	100
Chickpeas/Garbonzos	55
Chinese noodles	55
Cottage cheese	29
Croutons	28
Cucumber	3
Egg, chopped	110
Gelatin parfait	50
Granola	65
Green pepper	6
Lettuce	2
Onions, chopped	14
Pasta/Macaroni salad	93
Peaches	48
Peas	28
Sunflower seeds	160

calories

* Counts are based on one-quarter cup servings.

Alphabetical Chart
(for Hi-Low Comparison Charts, see pages 83 - 164)

SALAD DRESSINGS*

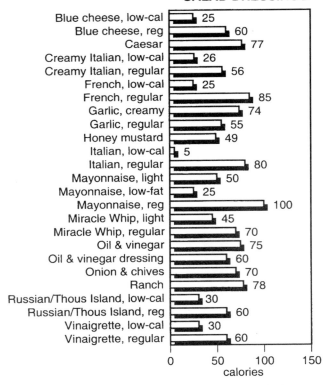

Dressing	calories
Blue cheese, low-cal	25
Blue cheese, reg	60
Caesar	77
Creamy Italian, low-cal	26
Creamy Italian, regular	56
French, low-cal	25
French, regular	85
Garlic, creamy	74
Garlic, regular	55
Honey mustard	49
Italian, low-cal	5
Italian, regular	80
Mayonnaise, light	50
Mayonnaise, low-fat	25
Mayonnaise, reg	100
Miracle Whip, light	45
Miracle Whip, regular	70
Oil & vinegar	75
Oil & vinegar dressing	60
Onion & chives	70
Ranch	78
Russian/Thous Island, low-cal	30
Russian/Thous Island, reg	60
Vinaigrette, low-cal	30
Vinaigrette, regular	60

* For ease of comparison, counts are based on single-tablespoon servings. Adjust counts to reflect quantities consumed.

SEAFOOD*, Part 1

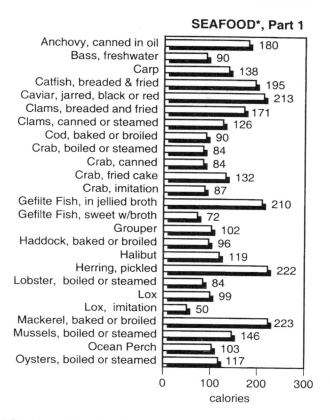

	calories
Anchovy, canned in oil	180
Bass, freshwater	90
Carp	138
Catfish, breaded & fried	195
Caviar, jarred, black or red	213
Clams, breaded and fried	171
Clams, canned or steamed	126
Cod, baked or broiled	90
Crab, boiled or steamed	84
Crab, canned	84
Crab, fried cake	132
Crab, imitation	87
Gefilte Fish, in jellied broth	210
Gefilte Fish, sweet w/broth	72
Grouper	102
Haddock, baked or broiled	96
Halibut	119
Herring, pickled	222
Lobster, boiled or steamed	84
Lox	99
Lox, imitation	50
Mackerel, baked or broiled	223
Mussels, boiled or steamed	146
Ocean Perch	103
Oysters, boiled or steamed	117

* Counts are based on 3-ounce servings. Canned seafood
items are assumed to be drained.

SEAFOOD*, Part 2

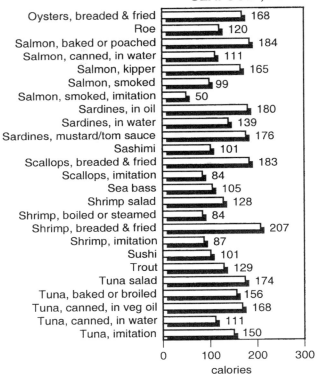

	calories
Oysters, breaded & fried	168
Roe	120
Salmon, baked or poached	184
Salmon, canned, in water	111
Salmon, kipper	165
Salmon, smoked	99
Salmon, smoked, imitation	50
Sardines, in oil	180
Sardines, in water	139
Sardines, mustard/tom sauce	176
Sashimi	101
Scallops, breaded & fried	183
Scallops, imitation	84
Sea bass	105
Shrimp salad	128
Shrimp, boiled or steamed	84
Shrimp, breaded & fried	207
Shrimp, imitation	87
Sushi	101
Trout	129
Tuna salad	174
Tuna, baked or broiled	156
Tuna, canned, in veg oil	168
Tuna, canned, in water	111
Tuna, imitation	150

* Counts are based on 3-ounce servings. Canned seafood
  items are assumed to be drained.

SNACK FOODS AND CHIPS: Part 1*

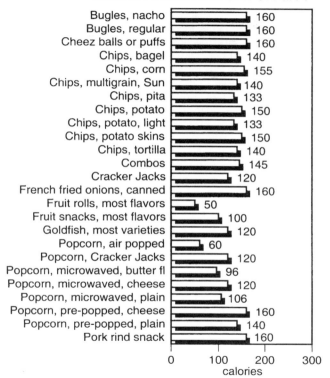

Food	calories
Bugles, nacho	160
Bugles, regular	160
Cheez balls or puffs	160
Chips, bagel	140
Chips, corn	155
Chips, multigrain, Sun	140
Chips, pita	133
Chips, potato	150
Chips, potato, light	133
Chips, potato skins	150
Chips, tortilla	140
Combos	145
Cracker Jacks	120
French fried onions, canned	160
Fruit rolls, most flavors	50
Fruit snacks, most flavors	100
Goldfish, most varieties	120
Popcorn, air popped	60
Popcorn, Cracker Jacks	120
Popcorn, microwaved, butter fl	96
Popcorn, microwaved, cheese	120
Popcorn, microwaved, plain	106
Popcorn, pre-popped, cheese	160
Popcorn, pre-popped, plain	140
Pork rind snack	160

* For ease of comparison, counts are based on one-ounce
servings. For popcorn, 1 ounce unpopped = 2 cups popped.
Adjust count to reflect amount consumed.

SNACK FOODS AND CHIPS: Part 2*

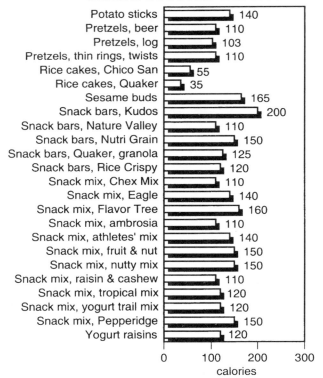

Food	calories
Potato sticks	140
Pretzels, beer	110
Pretzels, log	103
Pretzels, thin rings, twists	110
Rice cakes, Chico San	55
Rice cakes, Quaker	35
Sesame buds	165
Snack bars, Kudos	200
Snack bars, Nature Valley	110
Snack bars, Nutri Grain	150
Snack bars, Quaker, granola	125
Snack bars, Rice Crispy	120
Snack mix, Chex Mix	110
Snack mix, Eagle	140
Snack mix, Flavor Tree	160
Snack mix, ambrosia	110
Snack mix, athletes' mix	140
Snack mix, fruit & nut	150
Snack mix, nutty mix	150
Snack mix, raisin & cashew	110
Snack mix, tropical mix	120
Snack mix, yogurt trail mix	120
Snack mix, Pepperidge	150
Yogurt raisins	120

* For ease of comparison, counts are based on one-ounce
servings. For popcorn, 1 ounce unpopped = 2 cups popped.
Adjust count to reflect amount consumed.

Alphabetical Chart
(for Hi-Low Comparison Charts, see pages 83 - 164)

SOUP: Part 1

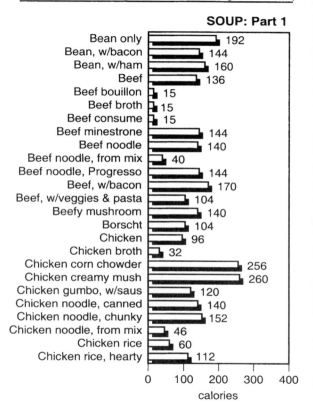

Soup	Calories
Bean only	192
Bean, w/bacon	144
Bean, w/ham	160
Beef	136
Beef bouillon	15
Beef broth	15
Beef consume	15
Beef minestrone	144
Beef noodle	140
Beef noodle, from mix	40
Beef noodle, Progresso	144
Beef, w/bacon	170
Beef, w/veggies & pasta	104
Beefy mushroom	140
Borscht	104
Chicken	96
Chicken broth	32
Chicken corn chowder	256
Chicken creamy mush	260
Chicken gumbo, w/saus	120
Chicken noodle, canned	140
Chicken noodle, chunky	152
Chicken noodle, from mix	46
Chicken rice	60
Chicken rice, hearty	112

calories (0, 100, 200, 300, 400)

* Counts are based on one-cup servings.

SOUP*, Part 2

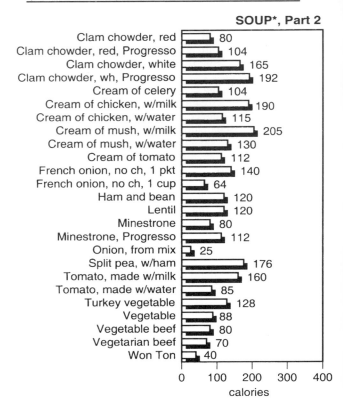

Soup	calories
Clam chowder, red	80
Clam chowder, red, Progresso	104
Clam chowder, white	165
Clam chowder, wh, Progresso	192
Cream of celery	104
Cream of chicken, w/milk	190
Cream of chicken, w/water	115
Cream of mush, w/milk	205
Cream of mush, w/water	130
Cream of tomato	112
French onion, no ch, 1 pkt	140
French onion, no ch, 1 cup	64
Ham and bean	120
Lentil	120
Minestrone	80
Minestrone, Progresso	112
Onion, from mix	25
Split pea, w/ham	176
Tomato, made w/milk	160
Tomato, made w/water	85
Turkey vegetable	128
Vegetable	88
Vegetable beef	80
Vegetarian beef	70
Won Ton	40

calories (0, 100, 200, 300, 400)

* Unless otherwise indicated, counts are based on one-cup
servings.

Sweets: CAKES*, Part 1

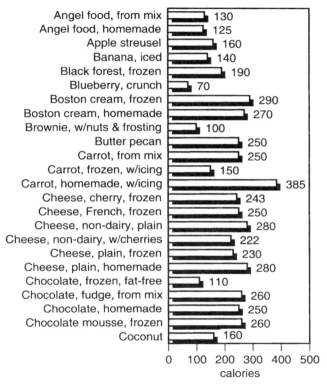

	calories
Angel food, from mix	130
Angel food, homemade	125
Apple streusel	160
Banana, iced	140
Black forest, frozen	190
Blueberry, crunch	70
Boston cream, frozen	290
Boston cream, homemade	270
Brownie, w/nuts & frosting	100
Butter pecan	250
Carrot, from mix	250
Carrot, frozen, w/icing	150
Carrot, homemade, w/icing	385
Cheese, cherry, frozen	243
Cheese, French, frozen	250
Cheese, non-dairy, plain	280
Cheese, non-dairy, w/cherries	222
Cheese, plain, frozen	230
Cheese, plain, homemade	280
Chocolate, frozen, fat-free	110
Chocolate, fudge, from mix	260
Chocolate, homemade	250
Chocolate mousse, frozen	260
Coconut	160

0   100   200   300   400   500
calories

* Counts are based on average-size pieces and slices,
  where appropriate, as indicated on package.

Sweets: CAKES*, Part 2

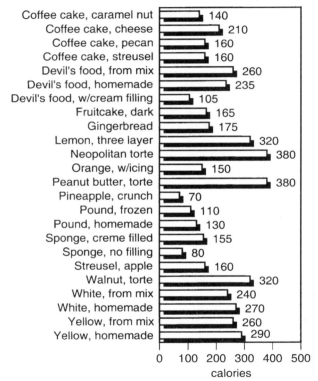

Cake	calories
Coffee cake, caramel nut	140
Coffee cake, cheese	210
Coffee cake, pecan	160
Coffee cake, streusel	160
Devil's food, from mix	260
Devil's food, homemade	235
Devil's food, w/cream filling	105
Fruitcake, dark	165
Gingerbread	175
Lemon, three layer	320
Neopolitan torte	380
Orange, w/icing	150
Peanut butter, torte	380
Pineapple, crunch	70
Pound, frozen	110
Pound, homemade	130
Sponge, creme filled	155
Sponge, no filling	80
Streusel, apple	160
Walnut, torte	320
White, from mix	240
White, homemade	270
Yellow, from mix	260
Yellow, homemade	290

* Counts are based on average-size pieces and slices,
  where appropriate, as indicated on package.

Alphabetical Chart
(for Hi-Low Comparison Charts, see pages 83 - 164)

Sweets: SNACK CAKES*

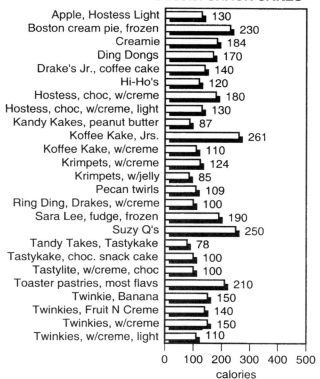

	calories
Apple, Hostess Light	130
Boston cream pie, frozen	230
Creamie	184
Ding Dongs	170
Drake's Jr., coffee cake	140
Hi-Ho's	120
Hostess, choc, w/creme	180
Hostess, choc, w/creme, light	130
Kandy Kakes, peanut butter	87
Koffee Kake, Jrs.	261
Koffee Kake, w/creme	110
Krimpets, w/creme	124
Krimpets, w/jelly	85
Pecan twirls	109
Ring Ding, Drakes, w/creme	100
Sara Lee, fudge, frozen	190
Suzy Q's	250
Tandy Takes, Tastykake	78
Tastykake, choc. snack cake	100
Tastylite, w/creme, choc	100
Toaster pastries, most flavs	210
Twinkie, Banana	150
Twinkies, Fruit N Creme	140
Twinkies, w/creme	150
Twinkies, w/creme, light	110

0   100   200   300   400   500
calories

* Counts are based on average-size pieces and slices,
where appropriate, as indicated on package.

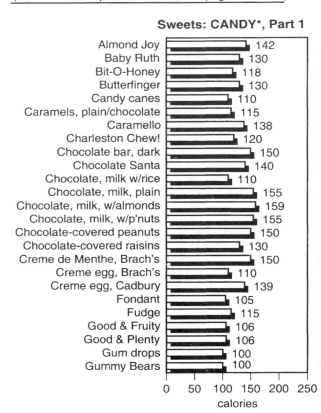

Sweets: CANDY*, Part 1

	calories
Almond Joy	142
Baby Ruth	130
Bit-O-Honey	118
Butterfinger	130
Candy canes	110
Caramels, plain/chocolate	115
Caramello	138
Charleston Chew!	120
Chocolate bar, dark	150
Chocolate Santa	140
Chocolate, milk w/rice	110
Chocolate, milk, plain	155
Chocolate, milk, w/almonds	159
Chocolate, milk, w/p'nuts	155
Chocolate-covered peanuts	150
Chocolate-covered raisins	130
Creme de Menthe, Brach's	150
Creme egg, Brach's	110
Creme egg, Cadbury	139
Fondant	105
Fudge	115
Good & Fruity	106
Good & Plenty	106
Gum drops	100
Gummy Bears	100

0   50   100   150   200   250
calories

* For ease of comparison, counts are based on one-ounce
servings. Adjust counts to reflect quantities consumed.

Sweets: CANDY*, Part 2

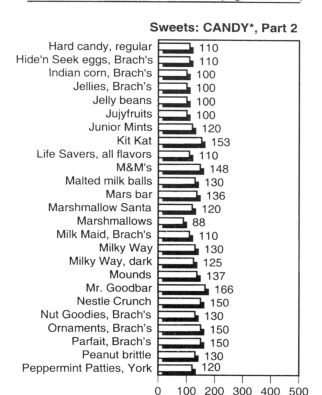

	calories
Hard candy, regular	110
Hide'n Seek eggs, Brach's	110
Indian corn, Brach's	100
Jellies, Brach's	100
Jelly beans	100
Jujyfruits	100
Junior Mints	120
Kit Kat	153
Life Savers, all flavors	110
M&M's	148
Malted milk balls	130
Mars bar	136
Marshmallow Santa	120
Marshmallows	88
Milk Maid, Brach's	110
Milky Way	130
Milky Way, dark	125
Mounds	137
Mr. Goodbar	166
Nestle Crunch	150
Nut Goodies, Brach's	130
Ornaments, Brach's	150
Parfait, Brach's	150
Peanut brittle	130
Peppermint Patties, York	120

* For ease of comparison, counts are based on one-ounce
servings. Adjust counts to reflect quantities consumed.

Sweets: CANDY*, Part 3

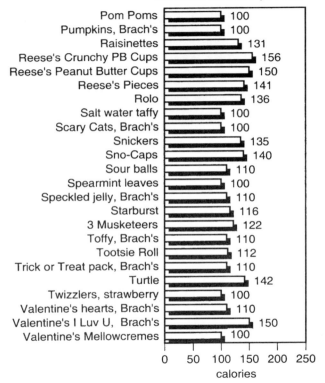

Candy	calories
Pom Poms	100
Pumpkins, Brach's	100
Raisinettes	131
Reese's Crunchy PB Cups	156
Reese's Peanut Butter Cups	150
Reese's Pieces	141
Rolo	136
Salt water taffy	100
Scary Cats, Brach's	100
Snickers	135
Sno-Caps	140
Sour balls	110
Spearmint leaves	100
Speckled jelly, Brach's	110
Starburst	116
3 Musketeers	122
Toffy, Brach's	110
Tootsie Roll	112
Trick or Treat pack, Brach's	110
Turtle	142
Twizzlers, strawberry	100
Valentine's hearts, Brach's	110
Valentine's I Luv U, Brach's	150
Valentine's Mellowcremes	100

calories (0 50 100 150 200 250)

* For ease of comparison, counts are based on one-ounce
servings. Adjust counts to reflect quantities consumed.

Sweets: COOKIES*, Part 1

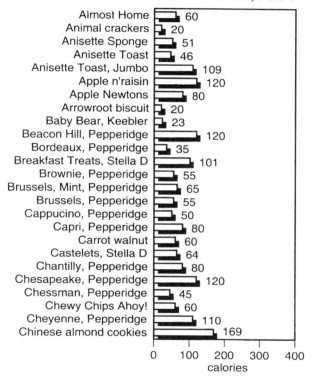

Cookie	Calories
Almost Home	60
Animal crackers	20
Anisette Sponge	51
Anisette Toast	46
Anisette Toast, Jumbo	109
Apple n'raisin	120
Apple Newtons	80
Arrowroot biscuit	20
Baby Bear, Keebler	23
Beacon Hill, Pepperidge	120
Bordeaux, Pepperidge	35
Breakfast Treats, Stella D	101
Brownie, Pepperidge	55
Brussels, Mint, Pepperidge	65
Brussels, Pepperidge	55
Cappucino, Pepperidge	50
Capri, Pepperidge	80
Carrot walnut	60
Castelets, Stella D	64
Chantilly, Pepperidge	80
Chesapeake, Pepperidge	120
Chessman, Pepperidge	45
Chewy Chips Ahoy!	60
Cheyenne, Pepperidge	110
Chinese almond cookies	169

calories (0, 100, 200, 300, 400)

* NOTE: For ease of comparison, counts are based on
single cookie servings. When more than one cookie is
consumed, counts should be adjusted accordingly.

Sweets: COOKIES*, Part 2

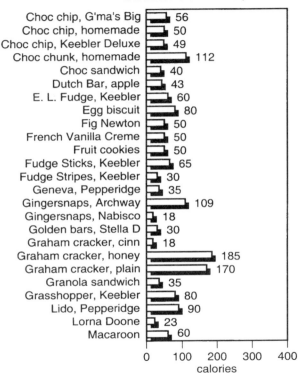

	calories
Choc chip, G'ma's Big	56
Choc chip, homemade	50
Choc chip, Keebler Deluxe	49
Choc chunk, homemade	112
Choc sandwich	40
Dutch Bar, apple	43
E. L. Fudge, Keebler	60
Egg biscuit	80
Fig Newton	50
French Vanilla Creme	50
Fruit cookies	50
Fudge Sticks, Keebler	65
Fudge Stripes, Keebler	30
Geneva, Pepperidge	35
Gingersnaps, Archway	109
Gingersnaps, Nabisco	18
Golden bars, Stella D	30
Graham cracker, cinn	18
Graham cracker, honey	185
Graham cracker, plain	170
Granola sandwich	35
Grasshopper, Keebler	80
Lido, Pepperidge	90
Lorna Doone	23
Macaroon	60

* NOTE: For ease of comparison, counts are based on
single cookie servings. When more than one cookie is
consumed, counts should be adjusted accordingly.

Sweets: COOKIES*, Part 3

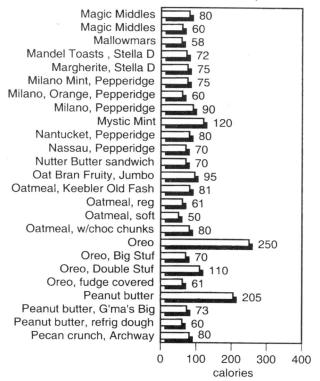

Cookie	calories
Magic Middles	80
Magic Middles	60
Mallowmars	58
Mandel Toasts , Stella D	72
Margherite, Stella D	75
Milano Mint, Pepperidge	75
Milano, Orange, Pepperidge	60
Milano, Pepperidge	90
Mystic Mint	120
Nantucket, Pepperidge	80
Nassau, Pepperidge	70
Nutter Butter sandwich	70
Oat Bran Fruity, Jumbo	95
Oatmeal, Keebler Old Fash	81
Oatmeal, reg	61
Oatmeal, soft	50
Oatmeal, w/choc chunks	80
Oreo	250
Oreo, Big Stuf	70
Oreo, Double Stuf	110
Oreo, fudge covered	61
Peanut butter	205
Peanut butter, G'ma's Big	73
Peanut butter, refrig dough	60
Pecan crunch, Archway	80

* NOTE: For ease of comparison, counts are based on
single cookie servings. When more than one cookie is
consumed, counts should be adjusted accordingly.

71

Sweets: COOKIES*, Part 4

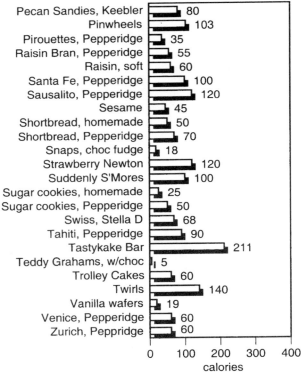

Cookie	calories
Pecan Sandies, Keebler	80
Pinwheels	103
Pirouettes, Pepperidge	35
Raisin Bran, Pepperidge	55
Raisin, soft	60
Santa Fe, Pepperidge	100
Sausalito, Pepperidge	120
Sesame	45
Shortbread, homemade	50
Shortbread, Pepperidge	70
Snaps, choc fudge	18
Strawberry Newton	120
Suddenly S'Mores	100
Sugar cookies, homemade	25
Sugar cookies, Pepperidge	50
Swiss, Stella D	68
Tahiti, Pepperidge	90
Tastykake Bar	211
Teddy Grahams, w/choc	5
Trolley Cakes	60
Twirls	140
Vanilla wafers	19
Venice, Pepperidge	60
Zurich, Peppridge	60

* NOTE: For ease of comparison, counts are based on
single cookie servings. When more than one cookie is
consumed, counts should be adjusted accordingly.

Sweets: DONUTS*

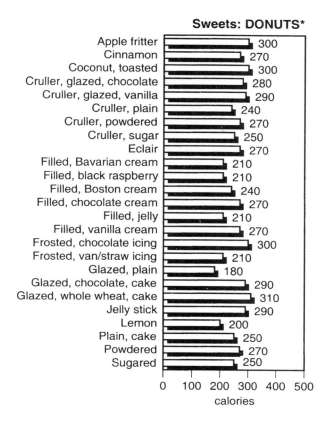

Donut	Calories
Apple fritter	300
Cinnamon	270
Coconut, toasted	300
Cruller, glazed, chocolate	280
Cruller, glazed, vanilla	290
Cruller, plain	240
Cruller, powdered	270
Cruller, sugar	250
Eclair	270
Filled, Bavarian cream	210
Filled, black raspberry	210
Filled, Boston cream	240
Filled, chocolate cream	270
Filled, jelly	210
Filled, vanilla cream	270
Frosted, chocolate icing	300
Frosted, van/straw icing	210
Glazed, plain	180
Glazed, chocolate, cake	290
Glazed, whole wheat, cake	310
Jelly stick	290
Lemon	200
Plain, cake	250
Powdered	270
Sugared	250

0   100   200   300   400   500
calories

* Counts are based on average-size donuts.

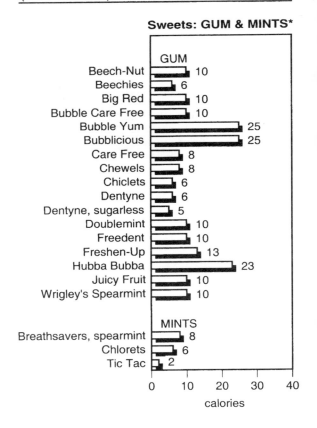

Sweets: GUM & MINTS*

GUM

Beech-Nut	10
Beechies	6
Big Red	10
Bubble Care Free	10
Bubble Yum	25
Bubblicious	25
Care Free	8
Chewels	8
Chiclets	6
Dentyne	6
Dentyne, sugarless	5
Doublemint	10
Freedent	10
Freshen-Up	13
Hubba Bubba	23
Juicy Fruit	10
Wrigley's Spearmint	10

MINTS

Breathsavers, spearmint	8
Chlorets	6
Tic Tac	2

0   10   20   30   40
calories

* Counts are based on single sticks or mints.

Sweets: ICE CREAM*

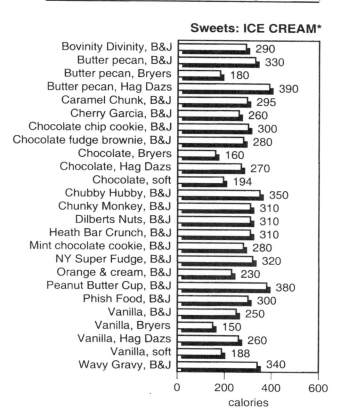

	calories
Bovinity Divinity, B&J	290
Butter pecan, B&J	330
Butter pecan, Bryers	180
Butter pecan, Hag Dazs	390
Caramel Chunk, B&J	295
Cherry Garcia, B&J	260
Chocolate chip cookie, B&J	300
Chocolate fudge brownie, B&J	280
Chocolate, Bryers	160
Chocolate, Hag Dazs	270
Chocolate, soft	194
Chubby Hubby, B&J	350
Chunky Monkey, B&J	310
Dilberts Nuts, B&J	310
Heath Bar Crunch, B&J	310
Mint chocolate cookie, B&J	280
NY Super Fudge, B&J	320
Orange & cream, B&J	230
Peanut Butter Cup, B&J	380
Phish Food, B&J	300
Vanilla, B&J	250
Vanilla, Bryers	150
Vanilla, Hag Dazs	260
Vanilla, soft	188
Wavy Gravy, B&J	340

* Counts are based on one-half cup servings. "B&J"
designates Ben & Jerry's brand.

Sweets: ICE CREAM CONES & BARS, ICE CREAM ALTERNATIVES AND PUDDINGS*

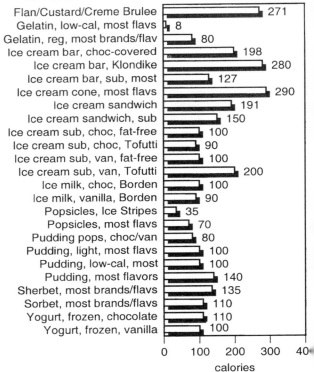

	calories
Flan/Custard/Creme Brulee	271
Gelatin, low-cal, most flavs	8
Gelatin, reg, most brands/flav	80
Ice cream bar, choc-covered	198
Ice cream bar, Klondike	280
Ice cream bar, sub, most	127
Ice cream cone, most flavs	290
Ice cream sandwich	191
Ice cream sandwich, sub	150
Ice cream sub, choc, fat-free	100
Ice cream sub, choc, Tofutti	90
Ice cream sub, van, fat-free	100
Ice cream sub, van, Tofutti	200
Ice milk, choc, Borden	100
Ice milk, vanilla, Borden	90
Popsicles, Ice Stripes	35
Popsicles, most flavs	70
Pudding pops, choc/van	80
Pudding, light, most flavs	100
Pudding, low-cal, most	100
Pudding, most flavors	140
Sherbet, most brands/flavs	135
Sorbet, most brands/flavs	110
Yogurt, frozen, chocolate	110
Yogurt, frozen, vanilla	100

0   100   200   300   40

calories

* Counts are based on average- or one-half cup serving.
"Sub" designates non-dairy, ice cream substitute.

Sweets: PIES*

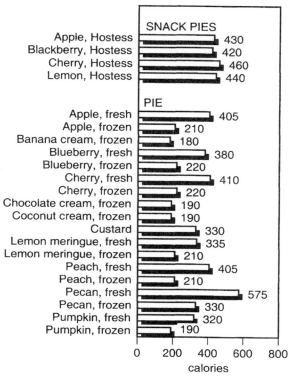

SNACK PIES

	calories
Apple, Hostess	430
Blackberry, Hostess	420
Cherry, Hostess	460
Lemon, Hostess	440

PIE

	calories
Apple, fresh	405
Apple, frozen	210
Banana cream, frozen	180
Blueberry, fresh	380
Blueberry, frozen	220
Cherry, fresh	410
Cherry, frozen	220
Chocolate cream, frozen	190
Coconut cream, frozen	190
Custard	330
Lemon meringue, fresh	335
Lemon meringue, frozen	210
Peach, fresh	405
Peach, frozen	210
Pecan, fresh	575
Pecan, frozen	330
Pumpkin, fresh	320
Pumpkin, frozen	190

0   200   400   600   800
calories

* Counts are based on average-size pieces and slices,
where appropriate, as indicated on package.

Sweets: SUGARS, SYRUPS, TOPPINGS AND JAMS*

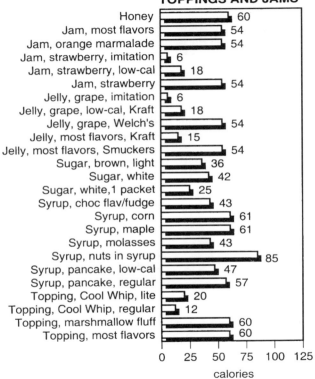

	calories
Honey	60
Jam, most flavors	54
Jam, orange marmalade	54
Jam, strawberry, imitation	6
Jam, strawberry, low-cal	18
Jam, strawberry	54
Jelly, grape, imitation	6
Jelly, grape, low-cal, Kraft	18
Jelly, grape, Welch's	54
Jelly, most flavors, Kraft	15
Jelly, most flavors, Smuckers	54
Sugar, brown, light	36
Sugar, white	42
Sugar, white, 1 packet	25
Syrup, choc flav/fudge	43
Syrup, corn	61
Syrup, maple	61
Syrup, molasses	43
Syrup, nuts in syrup	85
Syrup, pancake, low-cal	47
Syrup, pancake, regular	57
Topping, Cool Whip, lite	20
Topping, Cool Whip, regular	12
Topping, marshmallow fluff	60
Topping, most flavors	60

calories

* Counts are based on single-tablespoon servings. Jams and preserves can be assumed to have equal values.

VEGETABLES*, Part 1

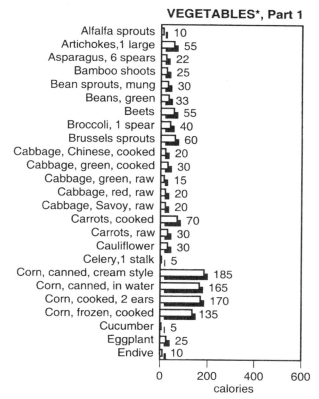

Vegetable	calories
Alfalfa sprouts	10
Artichokes, 1 large	55
Asparagus, 6 spears	22
Bamboo shoots	25
Bean sprouts, mung	30
Beans, green	33
Beets	55
Broccoli, 1 spear	40
Brussels sprouts	60
Cabbage, Chinese, cooked	20
Cabbage, green, cooked	30
Cabbage, green, raw	15
Cabbage, red, raw	20
Cabbage, Savoy, raw	20
Carrots, cooked	70
Carrots, raw	30
Cauliflower	30
Celery, 1 stalk	5
Corn, canned, cream style	185
Corn, canned, in water	165
Corn, cooked, 2 ears	170
Corn, frozen, cooked	135
Cucumber	5
Eggplant	25
Endive	10

0   200   400   600
calories

* Unless otherwise indicated, counts are based on one-cup
servings. For vegetable juices, see the Fruits & Juices
section.

VEGETABLES*, Part 2

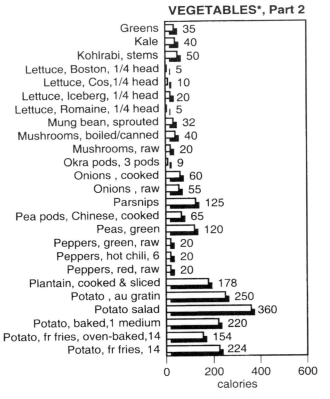

	calories
Greens	35
Kale	40
Kohlrabi, stems	50
Lettuce, Boston, 1/4 head	5
Lettuce, Cos, 1/4 head	10
Lettuce, Iceberg, 1/4 head	20
Lettuce, Romaine, 1/4 head	5
Mung bean, sprouted	32
Mushrooms, boiled/canned	40
Mushrooms, raw	20
Okra pods, 3 pods	9
Onions , cooked	60
Onions , raw	55
Parsnips	125
Pea pods, Chinese, cooked	65
Peas, green	120
Peppers, green, raw	20
Peppers, hot chili, 6	20
Peppers, red, raw	20
Plantain, cooked & sliced	178
Potato , au gratin	250
Potato salad	360
Potato, baked, 1 medium	220
Potato, fr fries, oven-baked, 14	154
Potato, fr fries, 14	224

0   200   400   600
calories

* Unless otherwise indicated, counts are based on one-cup
servings. For vegetable juices, see the Fruits & Juices
section.

VEGETABLES*, Part 3

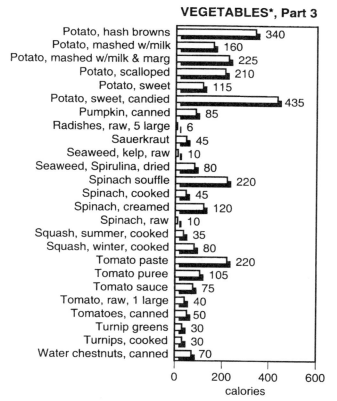

	calories
Potato, hash browns	340
Potato, mashed w/milk	160
Potato, mashed w/milk & marg	225
Potato, scalloped	210
Potato, sweet	115
Potato, sweet, candied	435
Pumpkin, canned	85
Radishes, raw, 5 large	6
Sauerkraut	45
Seaweed, kelp, raw	10
Seaweed, Spirulina, dried	80
Spinach souffle	220
Spinach, cooked	45
Spinach, creamed	120
Spinach, raw	10
Squash, summer, cooked	35
Squash, winter, cooked	80
Tomato paste	220
Tomato puree	105
Tomato sauce	75
Tomato, raw, 1 large	40
Tomatoes, canned	50
Turnip greens	30
Turnips, cooked	30
Water chestnuts, canned	70

0   200   400   600
calories

* Unless otherwise indicated, counts are based on one-cup
servings. For vegetable juices, see the Fruits & Juices
section.

VEGETARIAN CHOICES*

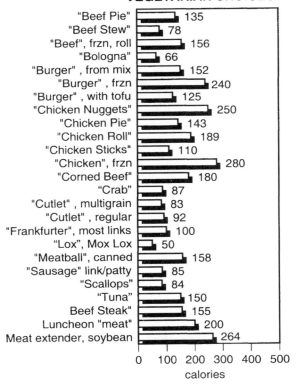

	calories
"Beef Pie"	135
"Beef Stew"	78
"Beef", frzn, roll	156
"Bologna"	66
"Burger", from mix	152
"Burger", frzn	240
"Burger", with tofu	125
"Chicken Nuggets"	250
"Chicken Pie"	143
"Chicken Roll"	189
"Chicken Sticks"	110
"Chicken", frzn	280
"Corned Beef"	180
"Crab"	87
"Cutlet", multigrain	83
"Cutlet", regular	92
"Frankfurter", most links	100
"Lox", Mox Lox	50
"Meatball", canned	158
"Sausage" link/patty	85
"Scallops"	84
"Tuna"	150
Beef Steak"	155
Luncheon "meat"	200
Meat extender, soybean	264

0   100   200   300   400   500
calories

* Made from tofu, textured vegetable protein or a combination of both. Counts are based on 3-ounce servings.

HI-LOW COMPARISON CHARTS

BEVERAGES*, Part 1

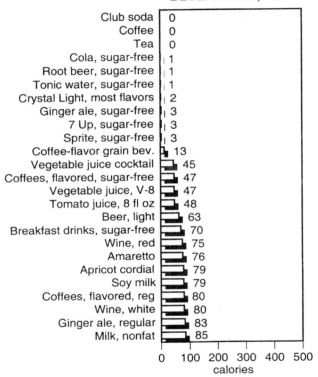

	calories
Club soda	0
Coffee	0
Tea	0
Cola, sugar-free	1
Root beer, sugar-free	1
Tonic water, sugar-free	1
Crystal Light, most flavors	2
Ginger ale, sugar-free	3
7 Up, sugar-free	3
Sprite, sugar-free	3
Coffee-flavor grain bev.	13
Vegetable juice cocktail	45
Coffees, flavored, sugar-free	47
Vegetable juice, V-8	47
Tomato juice, 8 fl oz	48
Beer, light	63
Breakfast drinks, sugar-free	70
Wine, red	75
Amaretto	76
Apricot cordial	79
Soy milk	79
Coffees, flavored, reg	80
Wine, white	80
Ginger ale, regular	83
Milk, nonfat	85

0   100   200   300   400   500
calories

* Counts for non-alcoholic drinks and beer are based on
8-fluid-ounce servings, for wine on 3 1/2-fluid-ounce
servings and, for hard liquor, on 1 1/2-fluid-ounce servings.

BEVERAGES*, Part 2

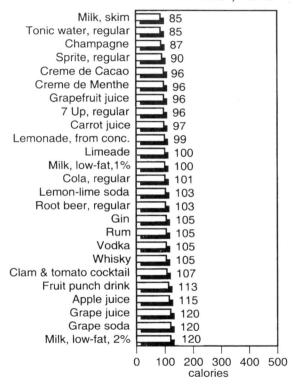

Beverage	calories
Milk, skim	85
Tonic water, regular	85
Champagne	87
Sprite, regular	90
Creme de Cacao	96
Creme de Menthe	96
Grapefruit juice	96
7 Up, regular	96
Carrot juice	97
Lemonade, from conc.	99
Limeade	100
Milk, low-fat, 1%	100
Cola, regular	101
Lemon-lime soda	103
Root beer, regular	103
Gin	105
Rum	105
Vodka	105
Whisky	105
Clam & tomato cocktail	107
Fruit punch drink	113
Apple juice	115
Grape juice	120
Grape soda	120
Milk, low-fat, 2%	120

0   100   200   300   400   500
calories

* Counts for non-alcoholic drinks and beer are based on
8-fluid-ounce servings, for wine on 3 1/2-fluid-ounce
servings and, for hard liquor, on 1 1/2-fluid-ounce servings.

BEVERAGES*, Part 3

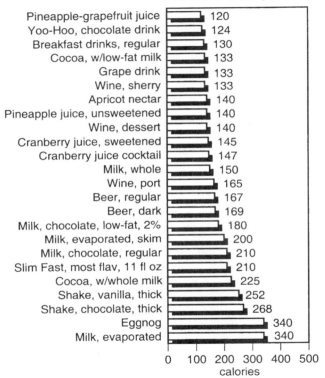

Beverage	calories
Pineapple-grapefruit juice	120
Yoo-Hoo, chocolate drink	124
Breakfast drinks, regular	130
Cocoa, w/low-fat milk	133
Grape drink	133
Wine, sherry	133
Apricot nectar	140
Pineapple juice, unsweetened	140
Wine, dessert	140
Cranberry juice, sweetened	145
Cranberry juice cocktail	147
Milk, whole	150
Wine, port	165
Beer, regular	167
Beer, dark	169
Milk, chocolate, low-fat, 2%	180
Milk, evaporated, skim	200
Milk, chocolate, regular	210
Slim Fast, most flav, 11 fl oz	210
Cocoa, w/whole milk	225
Shake, vanilla, thick	252
Shake, chocolate, thick	268
Eggnog	340
Milk, evaporated	340

0   100   200   300   400   500
calories

* Counts for non-alcoholic drinks and beer are based on
8-fluid-ounce servings, for wine on 3 1/2-fluid-ounce
servings and, for hard liquor, on 1 1/2-fluid-ounce servings.

Bread, Crackers, and Flours:
BAGELS*

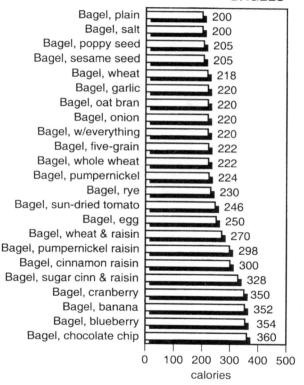

Bagel	calories
Bagel, plain	200
Bagel, salt	200
Bagel, poppy seed	205
Bagel, sesame seed	205
Bagel, wheat	218
Bagel, garlic	220
Bagel, oat bran	220
Bagel, onion	220
Bagel, w/everything	220
Bagel, five-grain	222
Bagel, whole wheat	222
Bagel, pumpernickel	224
Bagel, rye	230
Bagel, sun-dried tomato	246
Bagel, egg	250
Bagel, wheat & raisin	270
Bagel, pumpernickel raisin	298
Bagel, cinnamon raisin	300
Bagel, sugar cinn & raisin	328
Bagel, cranberry	350
Bagel, banana	352
Bagel, blueberry	354
Bagel, chocolate chip	360

calories

* Counts are based on one bagel, approximate weight:
3 ounces.

Bread, Crackers, and Flours:
BISCUITS, ROLLS & MUFFINS*

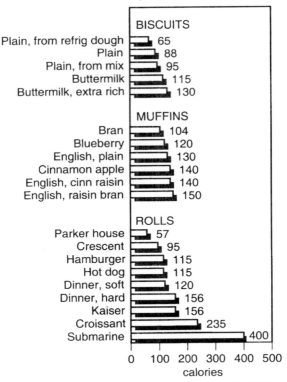

BISCUITS

Plain, from refrig dough	65
Plain	88
Plain, from mix	95
Buttermilk	115
Buttermilk, extra rich	130

MUFFINS

Bran	104
Blueberry	120
English, plain	130
Cinnamon apple	140
English, cinn raisin	140
English, raisin bran	150

ROLLS

Parker house	57
Crescent	95
Hamburger	115
Hot dog	115
Dinner, soft	120
Dinner, hard	156
Kaiser	156
Croissant	235
Submarine	400

0   100   200   300   400   500
calories

* Counts are based on single, average-size items. Average
sweet muffin is assumed to be 2 3/4 inches by 2 inches.
Average sweet and English muffin weight is 57 grams.

Bread, Crackers, and Flours:
BREAD*

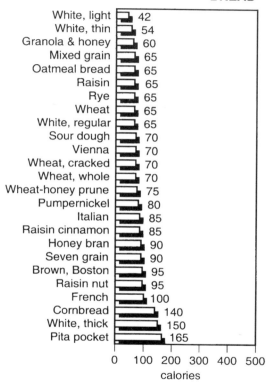

Bread	calories
White, light	42
White, thin	54
Granola & honey	60
Mixed grain	65
Oatmeal bread	65
Raisin	65
Rye	65
Wheat	65
White, regular	65
Sour dough	70
Vienna	70
Wheat, cracked	70
Wheat, whole	70
Wheat-honey prune	75
Pumpernickel	80
Italian	85
Raisin cinnamon	85
Honey bran	90
Seven grain	90
Brown, Boston	95
Raisin nut	95
French	100
Cornbread	140
White, thick	150
Pita pocket	165

0   100   200   300   400   500
calories

* Counts are based on single, average-size slices.

89

Bread, Crackers, and Flours:
CRACKERS*

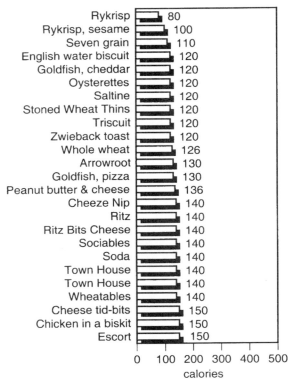

Cracker	calories
Rykrisp	80
Rykrisp, sesame	100
Seven grain	110
English water biscuit	120
Goldfish, cheddar	120
Oysterettes	120
Saltine	120
Stoned Wheat Thins	120
Triscuit	120
Zwieback toast	120
Whole wheat	126
Arrowroot	130
Goldfish, pizza	130
Peanut butter & cheese	136
Cheeze Nip	140
Ritz	140
Ritz Bits Cheese	140
Sociables	140
Soda	140
Town House	140
Town House	140
Wheatables	140
Cheese tid-bits	150
Chicken in a biskit	150
Escort	150

0   100   200   300   400   500
calories

* For ease of comparison, counts are based on one-ounce
servings. Adjust counts to reflect quantities consumed.

Bread, Crackers, and Flours:
DRY & CRISPY*

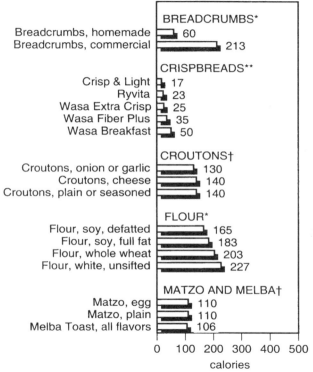

BREADCRUMBS*

Breadcrumbs, homemade — 60
Breadcrumbs, commercial — 213

CRISPBREADS**

Crisp & Light — 17
Ryvita — 23
Wasa Extra Crisp — 25
Wasa Fiber Plus — 35
Wasa Breakfast — 50

CROUTONS†

Croutons, onion or garlic — 130
Croutons, cheese — 140
Croutons, plain or seasoned — 140

FLOUR*

Flour, soy, defatted — 165
Flour, soy, full fat — 183
Flour, whole wheat — 203
Flour, white, unsifted — 227

MATZO AND MELBA†

Matzo, egg — 110
Matzo, plain — 110
Melba Toast, all flavors — 106

0   100   200   300   400   500
calories

* Counts are based on 1/2- cup servings.
Counts are based on single item.
† Counts are based on single-ounce servings.

Bread, Crackers, and Flours:
PANCAKES, STUFFING & MORE*

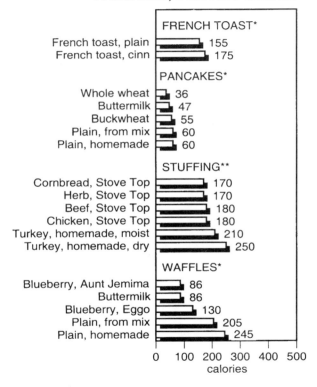

FRENCH TOAST*

French toast, plain	155
French toast, cinn	175

PANCAKES*

Whole wheat	36
Buttermilk	47
Buckwheat	55
Plain, from mix	60
Plain, homemade	60

STUFFING**

Cornbread, Stove Top	170
Herb, Stove Top	170
Beef, Stove Top	180
Chicken, Stove Top	180
Turkey, homemade, moist	210
Turkey, homemade, dry	250

WAFFLES*

Blueberry, Aunt Jemima	86
Buttermilk	86
Blueberry, Eggo	130
Plain, from mix	205
Plain, homemade	245

0   100   200   300   400   500
calories

* Counts are based on a single slice, waffle, or pancake.
** Counts are based on 1/2- cup servings after preparation.

CEREALS*, Part 1

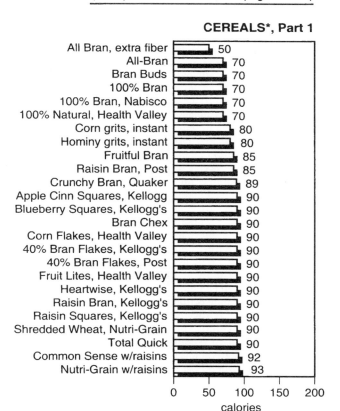

Cereal	calories
All Bran, extra fiber	50
All-Bran	70
Bran Buds	70
100% Bran	70
100% Bran, Nabisco	70
100% Natural, Health Valley	70
Corn grits, instant	80
Hominy grits, instant	80
Fruitful Bran	85
Raisin Bran, Post	85
Crunchy Bran, Quaker	89
Apple Cinn Squares, Kellogg	90
Blueberry Squares, Kellogg's	90
Bran Chex	90
Corn Flakes, Health Valley	90
40% Bran Flakes, Kellogg's	90
40% Bran Flakes, Post	90
Fruit Lites, Health Valley	90
Heartwise, Kellogg's	90
Raisin Bran, Kellogg's	90
Raisin Squares, Kellogg's	90
Shredded Wheat, Nutri-Grain	90
Total Quick	90
Common Sense w/raisins	92
Nutri-Grain w/raisins	93

* Counts are based on average-size servings (as indicated
on package) and without added milk.

CEREALS*, Part 2

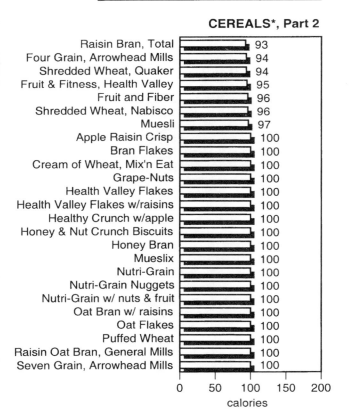

Cereal	calories
Raisin Bran, Total	93
Four Grain, Arrowhead Mills	94
Shredded Wheat, Quaker	94
Fruit & Fitness, Health Valley	95
Fruit and Fiber	96
Shredded Wheat, Nabisco	96
Muesli	97
Apple Raisin Crisp	100
Bran Flakes	100
Cream of Wheat, Mix'n Eat	100
Grape-Nuts	100
Health Valley Flakes	100
Health Valley Flakes w/raisins	100
Healthy Crunch w/apple	100
Honey & Nut Crunch Biscuits	100
Honey Bran	100
Mueslix	100
Nutri-Grain	100
Nutri-Grain Nuggets	100
Nutri-Grain w/ nuts & fruit	100
Oat Bran w/ raisins	100
Oat Flakes	100
Puffed Wheat	100
Raisin Oat Bran, General Mills	100
Seven Grain, Arrowhead Mills	100

0   50   100   150   200
calories

* Counts are based on average-size servings (as indicated
   on package) and without added milk.

CEREALS*, Part 3

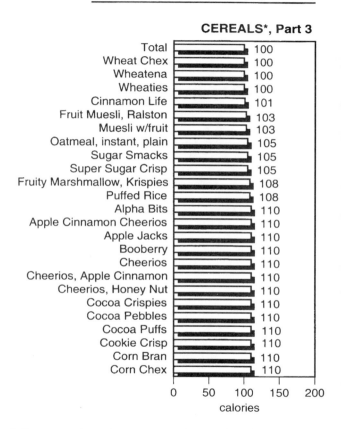

Cereal	calories
Total	100
Wheat Chex	100
Wheatena	100
Wheaties	100
Cinnamon Life	101
Fruit Muesli, Ralston	103
Muesli w/fruit	103
Oatmeal, instant, plain	105
Sugar Smacks	105
Super Sugar Crisp	105
Fruity Marshmallow, Krispies	108
Puffed Rice	108
Alpha Bits	110
Apple Cinnamon Cheerios	110
Apple Jacks	110
Booberry	110
Cheerios	110
Cheerios, Apple Cinnamon	110
Cheerios, Honey Nut	110
Cocoa Crispies	110
Cocoa Pebbles	110
Cocoa Puffs	110
Cookie Crisp	110
Corn Bran	110
Corn Chex	110

* Counts are based on average-size servings (as indicated on package) and without added milk.

CEREALS*, Part 4

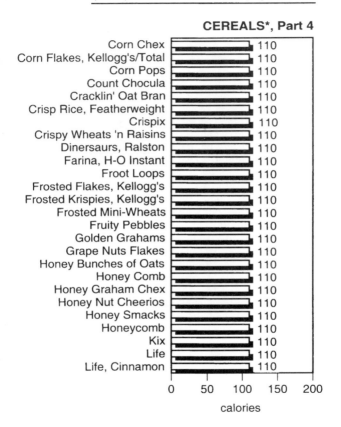

Cereal	calories
Corn Chex	110
Corn Flakes, Kellogg's/Total	110
Corn Pops	110
Count Chocula	110
Cracklin' Oat Bran	110
Crisp Rice, Featherweight	110
Crispix	110
Crispy Wheats 'n Raisins	110
Dinersaurs, Ralston	110
Farina, H-O Instant	110
Froot Loops	110
Frosted Flakes, Kellogg's	110
Frosted Krispies, Kellogg's	110
Frosted Mini-Wheats	110
Fruity Pebbles	110
Golden Grahams	110
Grape Nuts Flakes	110
Honey Bunches of Oats	110
Honey Comb	110
Honey Graham Chex	110
Honey Nut Cheerios	110
Honey Smacks	110
Honeycomb	110
Kix	110
Life	110
Life, Cinnamon	110

calories

* Counts are based on average-size servings (as indicated
on package) and without added milk.

CEREALS*, Part 5

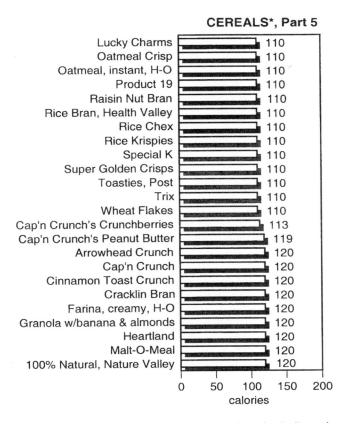

Cereal	calories
Lucky Charms	110
Oatmeal Crisp	110
Oatmeal, instant, H-O	110
Product 19	110
Raisin Nut Bran	110
Rice Bran, Health Valley	110
Rice Chex	110
Rice Krispies	110
Special K	110
Super Golden Crisps	110
Toasties, Post	110
Trix	110
Wheat Flakes	110
Cap'n Crunch's Crunchberries	113
Cap'n Crunch's Peanut Butter	119
Arrowhead Crunch	120
Cap'n Crunch	120
Cinnamon Toast Crunch	120
Cracklin Bran	120
Farina, creamy, H-O	120
Granola w/banana & almonds	120
Heartland	120
Malt-O-Meal	120
100% Natural, Nature Valley	120

0   50   100   150   200
calories

* Counts are based on average-size servings (as indicated
on package) and without added milk.

CEREALS*, Part 6

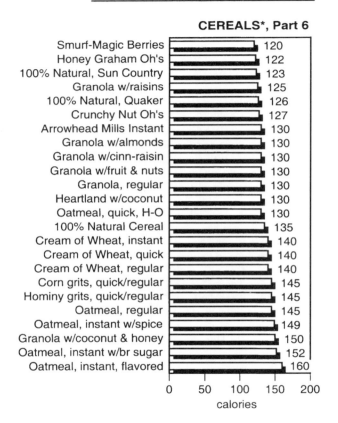

Cereal	calories
Smurf-Magic Berries	120
Honey Graham Oh's	122
100% Natural, Sun Country	123
Granola w/raisins	125
100% Natural, Quaker	126
Crunchy Nut Oh's	127
Arrowhead Mills Instant	130
Granola w/almonds	130
Granola w/cinn-raisin	130
Granola w/fruit & nuts	130
Granola, regular	130
Heartland w/coconut	130
Oatmeal, quick, H-O	130
100% Natural Cereal	135
Cream of Wheat, instant	140
Cream of Wheat, quick	140
Cream of Wheat, regular	140
Corn grits, quick/regular	145
Hominy grits, quick/regular	145
Oatmeal, regular	145
Oatmeal, instant w/spice	149
Granola w/coconut & honey	150
Oatmeal, instant w/br sugar	152
Oatmeal, instant, flavored	160

0   50   100   150   200
calories

* Counts are based on average-size servings (as indicated
on package) and without added milk.

COMBINED AND FROZEN FOODS*, Part 1

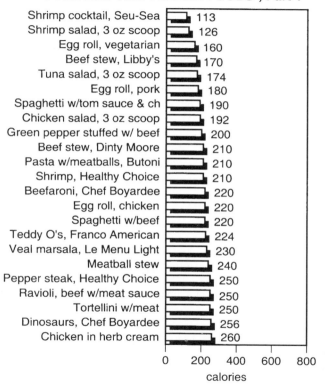

	calories
Shrimp cocktail, Seu-Sea	113
Shrimp salad, 3 oz scoop	126
Egg roll, vegetarian	160
Beef stew, Libby's	170
Tuna salad, 3 oz scoop	174
Egg roll, pork	180
Spaghetti w/tom sauce & ch	190
Chicken salad, 3 oz scoop	192
Green pepper stuffed w/ beef	200
Beef stew, Dinty Moore	210
Pasta w/meatballs, Butoni	210
Shrimp, Healthy Choice	210
Beefaroni, Chef Boyardee	220
Egg roll, chicken	220
Spaghetti w/beef	220
Teddy O's, Franco American	224
Veal marsala, Le Menu Light	230
Meatball stew	240
Pepper steak, Healthy Choice	250
Ravioli, beef w/meat sauce	250
Tortellini w/meat	250
Dinosaurs, Chef Boyardee	256
Chicken in herb cream	260

0   200   400   600   800
calories

* Counts are based on average-size servings as indicated
on package. Adjust count to reflect amount consumed.

COMBINED AND FROZEN FOODS*, Part 2

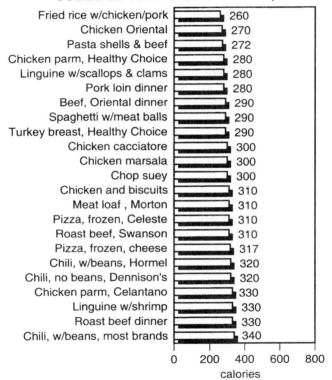

Food	calories
Fried rice w/chicken/pork	260
Chicken Oriental	270
Pasta shells & beef	272
Chicken parm, Healthy Choice	280
Linguine w/scallops & clams	280
Pork loin dinner	280
Beef, Oriental dinner	290
Spaghetti w/meat balls	290
Turkey breast, Healthy Choice	290
Chicken cacciatore	300
Chicken marsala	300
Chop suey	300
Chicken and biscuits	310
Meat loaf , Morton	310
Pizza, frozen, Celeste	310
Roast beef, Swanson	310
Pizza, frozen, cheese	317
Chili, w/beans, Hormel	320
Chili, no beans, Dennison's	320
Chicken parm, Celantano	330
Linguine w/shrimp	330
Roast beef dinner	330
Chili, w/beans, most brands	340

calories: 0   200   400   600   800

* Counts are based on average-size servings as indicated
on package. Adjust count to reflect amount consumed.

COMBINED AND FROZEN FOODS*, Part 3

Food	calories
Chopped sirloin	340
Crabs, devilled, 2	340
Chicken a la King	346
Fettuccini w/meat sauce	348
Pizza, french bread, pepperoni	350
Welsh Rarebit	350
Fettuccini alfredo	360
Ham & cheese pocket, frozen	360
Meat loaf , Swanson	360
Pizza pocket w/sausage	360
Chicken chow mein	370
Chicken pot pie, Swanson	370
Macaroni & beef	370
Lobster Newburg	380
Pizza, frozen, ch & pepperoni	380
Cinnamon swirls w/sausage	390
Manicotti, three cheese	390
Turkey dinner, most brands	390
Veal parmigiana, Le Menu	390
Chicken dinner, fried	400
Ham steak	400
Salisbury steak, Swanson	400
Chili, no beans, Hormel	413

calories (0 200 400 600 800)

* Counts are based on average-size servings as indicated
on package. Adjust count to reflect amount consumed.

COMBINED AND FROZEN FOODS*, Part 4

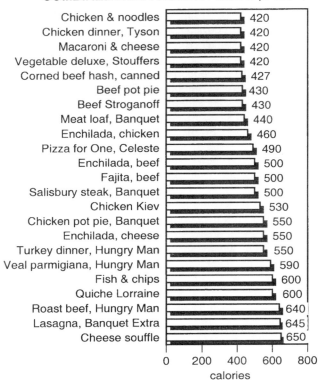

Food	calories
Chicken & noodles	420
Chicken dinner, Tyson	420
Macaroni & cheese	420
Vegetable deluxe, Stouffers	420
Corned beef hash, canned	427
Beef pot pie	430
Beef Stroganoff	430
Meat loaf, Banquet	440
Enchilada, chicken	460
Pizza for One, Celeste	490
Enchilada, beef	500
Fajita, beef	500
Salisbury steak, Banquet	500
Chicken Kiev	530
Chicken pot pie, Banquet	550
Enchilada, cheese	550
Turkey dinner, Hungry Man	550
Veal parmigiana, Hungry Man	590
Fish & chips	600
Quiche Lorraine	600
Roast beef, Hungry Man	640
Lasagna, Banquet Extra	645
Cheese souffle	650

* Counts are based on average-size servings as indicated
on package. Adjust count to reflect amount consumed.

Dairy: CHEESE (HARD & SEMI-SOFT)*

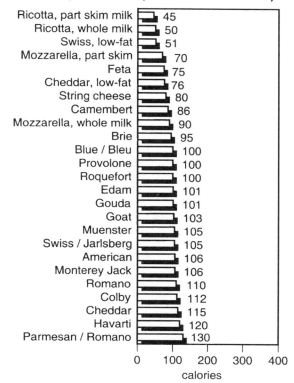

Cheese	calories
Ricotta, part skim milk	45
Ricotta, whole milk	50
Swiss, low-fat	51
Mozzarella, part skim	70
Feta	75
Cheddar, low-fat	76
String cheese	80
Camembert	86
Mozzarella, whole milk	90
Brie	95
Blue / Bleu	100
Provolone	100
Roquefort	100
Edam	101
Gouda	101
Goat	103
Muenster	105
Swiss / Jarlsberg	105
American	106
Monterey Jack	106
Romano	110
Colby	112
Cheddar	115
Havarti	120
Parmesan / Romano	130

* Counts are based on one-ounce servings. Adjust count to
  reflect amount consumed.

Dairy: CHEESES (SOFT), CREAMS & SUBSTITUTES*

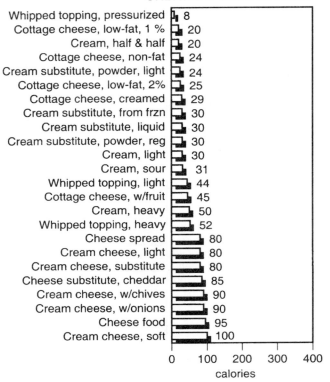

	calories
Whipped topping, pressurized	8
Cottage cheese, low-fat, 1 %	20
Cream, half & half	20
Cottage cheese, non-fat	24
Cream substitute, powder, light	24
Cottage cheese, low-fat, 2%	25
Cottage cheese, creamed	29
Cream substitute, from frzn	30
Cream substitute, liquid	30
Cream substitute, powder, reg	30
Cream, light	30
Cream, sour	31
Whipped topping, light	44
Cottage cheese, w/fruit	45
Cream, heavy	50
Whipped topping, heavy	52
Cheese spread	80
Cream cheese, light	80
Cream cheese, substitute	80
Cheese substitute, cheddar	85
Cream cheese, w/chives	90
Cream cheese, w/onions	90
Cheese food	95
Cream cheese, soft	100

0   100   200   300   400
calories

* Counts are based on one-ounce servings of soft cheese
or one tablespoon of cream or whipped topping.

Dairy: EGGS, MILK, YOGURT & SHAKES*

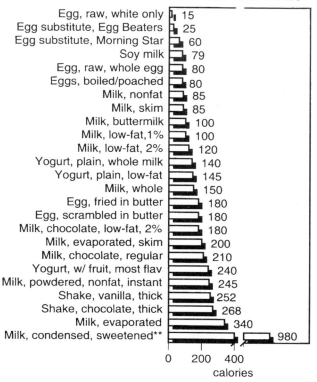

Item	calories
Egg, raw, white only	15
Egg substitute, Egg Beaters	25
Egg substitute, Morning Star	60
Soy milk	79
Egg, raw, whole egg	80
Eggs, boiled/poached	80
Milk, nonfat	85
Milk, skim	85
Milk, buttermilk	100
Milk, low-fat, 1%	100
Milk, low-fat, 2%	120
Yogurt, plain, whole milk	140
Yogurt, plain, low-fat	145
Milk, whole	150
Egg, fried in butter	180
Egg, scrambled in butter	180
Milk, chocolate, low-fat, 2%	180
Milk, evaporated, skim	200
Milk, chocolate, regular	210
Yogurt, w/ fruit, most flav	240
Milk, powdered, nonfat, instant	245
Shake, vanilla, thick	252
Shake, chocolate, thick	268
Milk, evaporated	340
Milk, condensed, sweetened**	980

0   200   400

calories

* Counts are based on one egg or equivalent egg substitute or 8 fluid ounces of milk, yogurt, or shake.

** High count for this item requires break in bar.

Dining Out: ASIAN*

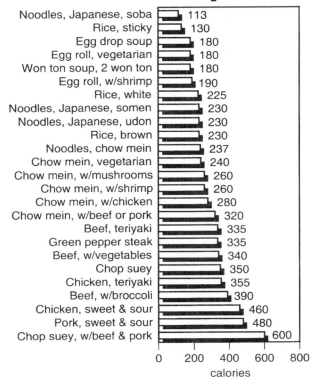

	calories
Noodles, Japanese, soba	113
Rice, sticky	130
Egg drop soup	180
Egg roll, vegetarian	180
Won ton soup, 2 won ton	180
Egg roll, w/shrimp	190
Rice, white	225
Noodles, Japanese, somen	230
Noodles, Japanese, udon	230
Rice, brown	230
Noodles, chow mein	237
Chow mein, vegetarian	240
Chow mein, w/mushrooms	260
Chow mein, w/shrimp	260
Chow mein, w/chicken	280
Chow mein, w/beef or pork	320
Beef, teriyaki	335
Green pepper steak	335
Beef, w/vegetables	340
Chop suey	350
Chicken, teriyaki	355
Beef, w/broccoli	390
Chicken, sweet & sour	460
Pork, sweet & sour	480
Chop suey, w/beef & pork	600

* Counts based on average-sized servings (for main dishes,
1 1/2 - 2 cups). Counts for main dishes include rice.

Dining Out: DELICATESSEN*

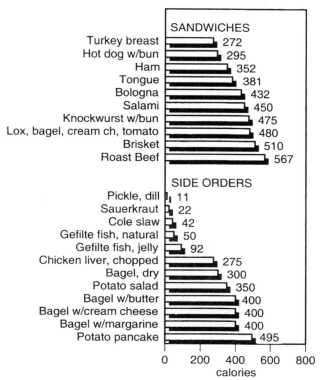

SANDWICHES

	calories
Turkey breast	272
Hot dog w/bun	295
Ham	352
Tongue	381
Bologna	432
Salami	450
Knockwurst w/bun	475
Lox, bagel, cream ch, tomato	480
Brisket	510
Roast Beef	567

SIDE ORDERS

	calories
Pickle, dill	11
Sauerkraut	22
Cole slaw	42
Gefilte fish, natural	50
Gefilte fish, jelly	92
Chicken liver, chopped	275
Bagel, dry	300
Potato salad	350
Bagel w/butter	400
Bagel w/cream cheese	400
Bagel w/margarine	400
Potato pancake	495

0   200   400   600   800
calories

* Unless otherwise indicated, counts based on average-
size servings or sandwiches. Sandwich counts assume
white or rye bread.

Dining Out: FRENCH AND
OTHER INTERNATIONAL DISHES*

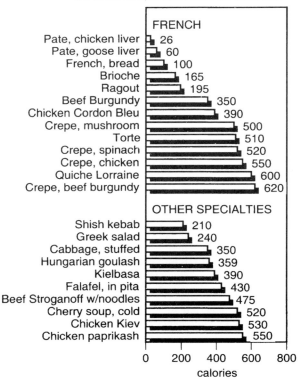

FRENCH

	calories
Pate, chicken liver	26
Pate, goose liver	60
French, bread	100
Brioche	165
Ragout	195
Beef Burgundy	350
Chicken Cordon Bleu	390
Crepe, mushroom	500
Torte	510
Crepe, spinach	520
Crepe, chicken	550
Quiche Lorraine	600
Crepe, beef burgundy	620

OTHER SPECIALTIES

	calories
Shish kebab	210
Greek salad	240
Cabbage, stuffed	350
Hungarian goulash	359
Kielbasa	390
Falafel, in pita	430
Beef Stroganoff w/noodles	475
Cherry soup, cold	520
Chicken Kiev	530
Chicken paprikash	550

0   200   400   600   800
calories

* Counts based on average-sized servings (for main dishes,
1 1/2 - 2 cups).

Dining Out: ITALIAN*

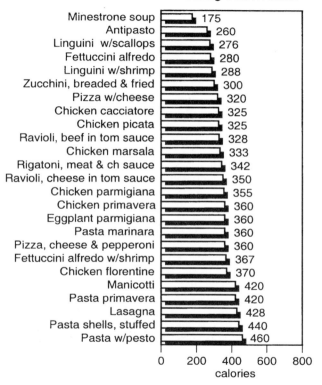

Food	Calories
Minestrone soup	175
Antipasto	260
Linguini w/scallops	276
Fettuccini alfredo	280
Linguini w/shrimp	288
Zucchini, breaded & fried	300
Pizza w/cheese	320
Chicken cacciatore	325
Chicken picata	325
Ravioli, beef in tom sauce	328
Chicken marsala	333
Rigatoni, meat & ch sauce	342
Ravioli, cheese in tom sauce	350
Chicken parmigiana	355
Chicken primavera	360
Eggplant parmigiana	360
Pasta marinara	360
Pizza, cheese & pepperoni	360
Fettuccini alfredo w/shrimp	367
Chicken florentine	370
Manicotti	420
Pasta primavera	420
Lasagna	428
Pasta shells, stuffed	440
Pasta w/pesto	460

calories: 0   200   400   600   800

* Counts are based on average-sized servings (1 1/2 - 2 cups); for pizza, on 1/6 medium or 1/8 large pizza).

Dining Out: MEXICAN*

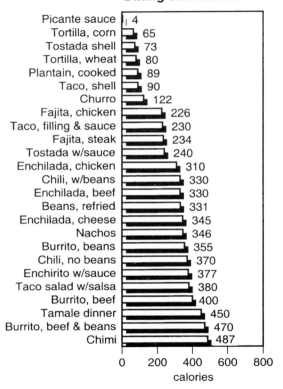

	calories
Picante sauce	4
Tortilla, corn	65
Tostada shell	73
Tortilla, wheat	80
Plantain, cooked	89
Taco, shell	90
Churro	122
Fajita, chicken	226
Taco, filling & sauce	230
Fajita, steak	234
Tostada w/sauce	240
Enchilada, chicken	310
Chili, w/beans	330
Enchilada, beef	330
Beans, refried	331
Enchilada, cheese	345
Nachos	346
Burrito, beans	355
Chili, no beans	370
Enchirito w/sauce	377
Taco salad w/salsa	380
Burrito, beef	400
Tamale dinner	450
Burrito, beef & beans	470
Chimi	487

calories

* Counts based on average-sized servings (for main dishes,
1 1/2 - 2 cups).

Hi-Low Comparison Chart
(for Alphabetical Charts, see pages 1 - 82)

Fast Food: ARBY'S*

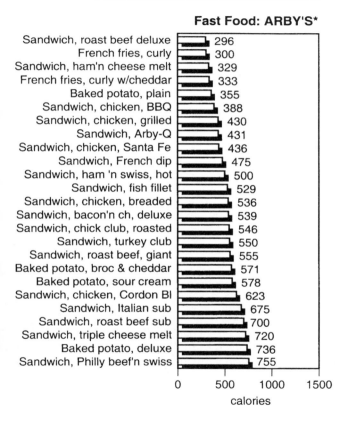

Item	Calories
Sandwich, roast beef deluxe	296
French fries, curly	300
Sandwich, ham'n cheese melt	329
French fries, curly w/cheddar	333
Baked potato, plain	355
Sandwich, chicken, BBQ	388
Sandwich, chicken, grilled	430
Sandwich, Arby-Q	431
Sandwich, chicken, Santa Fe	436
Sandwich, French dip	475
Sandwich, ham 'n swiss, hot	500
Sandwich, fish fillet	529
Sandwich, chicken, breaded	536
Sandwich, bacon'n ch, deluxe	539
Sandwich, chick club, roasted	546
Sandwich, turkey club	550
Sandwich, roast beef, giant	555
Baked potato, broc & cheddar	571
Baked potato, sour cream	578
Sandwich, chicken, Cordon Bl	623
Sandwich, Italian sub	675
Sandwich, roast beef sub	700
Sandwich, triple cheese melt	720
Baked potato, deluxe	736
Sandwich, Philly beef'n swiss	755

calories: 0   500   1000   1500

* Unless otherwise indicated, counts are based on average-size servings.

111

Fast Food: BOSTON MARKET*

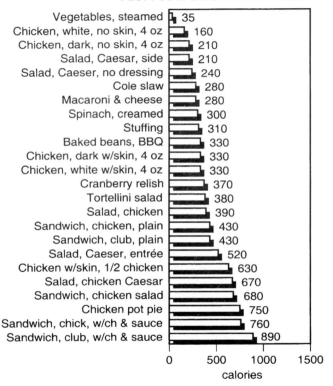

Item	calories
Vegetables, steamed	35
Chicken, white, no skin, 4 oz	160
Chicken, dark, no skin, 4 oz	210
Salad, Caesar, side	210
Salad, Caeser, no dressing	240
Cole slaw	280
Macaroni & cheese	280
Spinach, creamed	300
Stuffing	310
Baked beans, BBQ	330
Chicken, dark w/skin, 4 oz	330
Chicken, white w/skin, 4 oz	330
Cranberry relish	370
Tortellini salad	380
Salad, chicken	390
Sandwich, chicken, plain	430
Sandwich, club, plain	430
Salad, Caeser, entrée	520
Chicken w/skin, 1/2 chicken	630
Salad, chicken Caesar	670
Sandwich, chicken salad	680
Chicken pot pie	750
Sandwich, chick, w/ch & sauce	760
Sandwich, club, w/ch & sauce	890

*   Unless otherwise indicated, counts are based on average-
    size servings.

Hi-Low Comparison Chart
(for Alphabetical Charts, see pages 1 - 82)

Fast Food: BURGER KING*

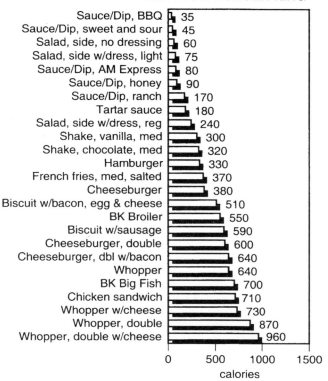

Item	calories
Sauce/Dip, BBQ	35
Sauce/Dip, sweet and sour	45
Salad, side, no dressing	60
Salad, side w/dress, light	75
Sauce/Dip, AM Express	80
Sauce/Dip, honey	90
Sauce/Dip, ranch	170
Tartar sauce	180
Salad, side w/dress, reg	240
Shake, vanilla, med	300
Shake, chocolate, med	320
Hamburger	330
French fries, med, salted	370
Cheeseburger	380
Biscuit w/bacon, egg & cheese	510
BK Broiler	550
Biscuit w/sausage	590
Cheeseburger, double	600
Cheeseburger, dbl w/bacon	640
Whopper	640
BK Big Fish	700
Chicken sandwich	710
Whopper w/cheese	730
Whopper, double	870
Whopper, double w/cheese	960

calories: 0   500   1000   1500

* Unless otherwise indicated, counts are based on average-size servings.

Fast Food: HARDEE'S*

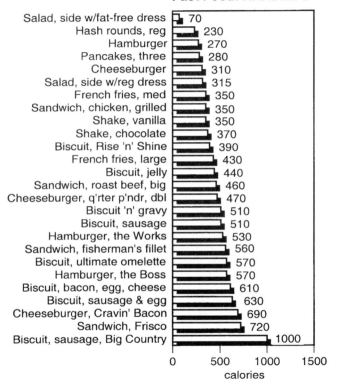

Item	calories
Salad, side w/fat-free dress	70
Hash rounds, reg	230
Hamburger	270
Pancakes, three	280
Cheeseburger	310
Salad, side w/reg dress	315
French fries, med	350
Sandwich, chicken, grilled	350
Shake, vanilla	350
Shake, chocolate	370
Biscuit, Rise 'n' Shine	390
French fries, large	430
Biscuit, jelly	440
Sandwich, roast beef, big	460
Cheeseburger, q'rter p'ndr, dbl	470
Biscuit 'n' gravy	510
Biscuit, sausage	510
Hamburger, the Works	530
Sandwich, fisherman's fillet	560
Biscuit, ultimate omelette	570
Hamburger, the Boss	570
Biscuit, bacon, egg, cheese	610
Biscuit, sausage & egg	630
Cheeseburger, Cravin' Bacon	690
Sandwich, Frisco	720
Biscuit, sausage, Big Country	1000

0   500   1000   1500
calories

* Unless otherwise indicated, counts are based on average-
size servings.

114

Fast Food: JACK IN THE BOX*

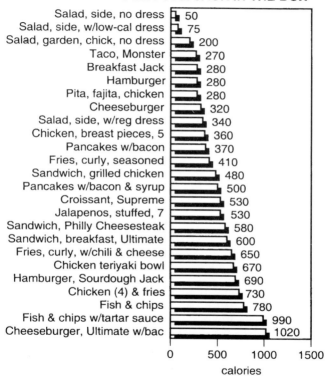

Item	calories
Salad, side, no dress	50
Salad, side, w/low-cal dress	75
Salad, garden, chick, no dress	200
Taco, Monster	270
Breakfast Jack	280
Hamburger	280
Pita, fajita, chicken	280
Cheeseburger	320
Salad, side, w/reg dress	340
Chicken, breast pieces, 5	360
Pancakes w/bacon	370
Fries, curly, seasoned	410
Sandwich, grilled chicken	480
Pancakes w/bacon & syrup	500
Croissant, Supreme	530
Jalapenos, stuffed, 7	530
Sandwich, Philly Cheesesteak	580
Sandwich, breakfast, Ultimate	600
Fries, curly, w/chili & cheese	650
Chicken teriyaki bowl	670
Hamburger, Sourdough Jack	690
Chicken (4) & fries	730
Fish & chips	780
Fish & chips w/tartar sauce	990
Cheeseburger, Ultimate w/bac	1020

0   500   1000   1500
calories

* Unless otherwise indicated, counts are based on average-
size servings.

Fast Food: KFC*

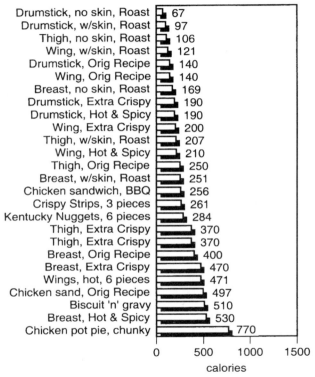

Food	calories
Drumstick, no skin, Roast	67
Drumstick, w/skin, Roast	97
Thigh, no skin, Roast	106
Wing, w/skin, Roast	121
Drumstick, Orig Recipe	140
Wing, Orig Recipe	140
Breast, no skin, Roast	169
Drumstick, Extra Crispy	190
Drumstick, Hot & Spicy	190
Wing, Extra Crispy	200
Thigh, w/skin, Roast	207
Wing, Hot & Spicy	210
Thigh, Orig Recipe	250
Breast, w/skin, Roast	251
Chicken sandwich, BBQ	256
Crispy Strips, 3 pieces	261
Kentucky Nuggets, 6 pieces	284
Thigh, Extra Crispy	370
Thigh, Extra Crispy	370
Breast, Orig Recipe	400
Breast, Extra Crispy	470
Wings, hot, 6 pieces	471
Chicken sand, Orig Recipe	497
Biscuit 'n' gravy	510
Breast, Hot & Spicy	530
Chicken pot pie, chunky	770

* Unless otherwise indicated, counts are based on average-size servings.

116

Fast Food: MC DONALD'S*

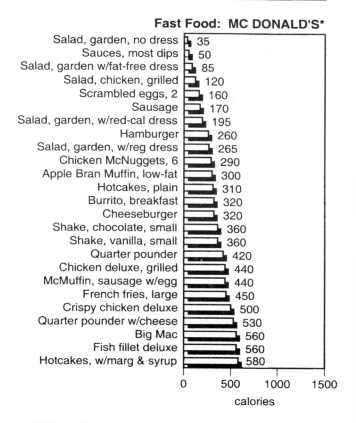

Food	calories
Salad, garden, no dress	35
Sauces, most dips	50
Salad, garden w/fat-free dress	85
Salad, chicken, grilled	120
Scrambled eggs, 2	160
Sausage	170
Salad, garden, w/red-cal dress	195
Hamburger	260
Salad, garden, w/reg dress	265
Chicken McNuggets, 6	290
Apple Bran Muffin, low-fat	300
Hotcakes, plain	310
Burrito, breakfast	320
Cheeseburger	320
Shake, chocolate, small	360
Shake, vanilla, small	360
Quarter pounder	420
Chicken deluxe, grilled	440
McMuffin, sausage w/egg	440
French fries, large	450
Crispy chicken deluxe	500
Quarter pounder w/cheese	530
Big Mac	560
Fish fillet deluxe	560
Hotcakes, w/marg & syrup	580

calories

* Unless otherwise indicated, counts are based on average-size servings.

117

Fast Food: PIZZA HUT*

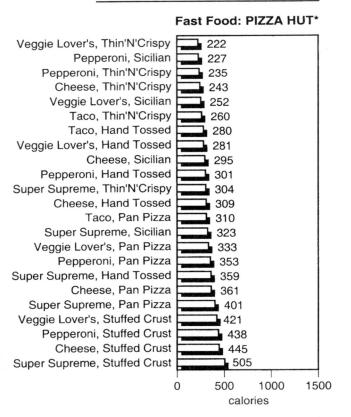

	calories
Veggie Lover's, Thin'N'Crispy	222
Pepperoni, Sicilian	227
Pepperoni, Thin'N'Crispy	235
Cheese, Thin'N'Crispy	243
Veggie Lover's, Sicilian	252
Taco, Thin'N'Crispy	260
Taco, Hand Tossed	280
Veggie Lover's, Hand Tossed	281
Cheese, Sicilian	295
Pepperoni, Hand Tossed	301
Super Supreme, Thin'N'Crispy	304
Cheese, Hand Tossed	309
Taco, Pan Pizza	310
Super Supreme, Sicilian	323
Veggie Lover's, Pan Pizza	333
Pepperoni, Pan Pizza	353
Super Supreme, Hand Tossed	359
Cheese, Pan Pizza	361
Super Supreme, Pan Pizza	401
Veggie Lover's, Stuffed Crust	421
Pepperoni, Stuffed Crust	438
Cheese, Stuffed Crust	445
Super Supreme, Stuffed Crust	505

* Unless otherwise indicated, counts are based on average-size servings.

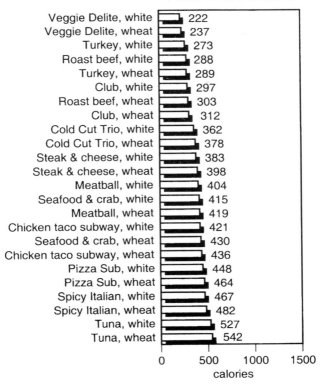

Hi-Low Comparison Chart
(for Alphabetical Charts, see pages 1 - 82)

Fast Food: SUBWAY*

Item	calories
Veggie Delite, white	222
Veggie Delite, wheat	237
Turkey, white	273
Roast beef, white	288
Turkey, wheat	289
Club, white	297
Roast beef, wheat	303
Club, wheat	312
Cold Cut Trio, white	362
Cold Cut Trio, wheat	378
Steak & cheese, white	383
Steak & cheese, wheat	398
Meatball, white	404
Seafood & crab, white	415
Meatball, wheat	419
Chicken taco subway, white	421
Seafood & crab, wheat	430
Chicken taco subway, wheat	436
Pizza Sub, white	448
Pizza Sub, wheat	464
Spicy Italian, white	467
Spicy Italian, wheat	482
Tuna, white	527
Tuna, wheat	542

calories (0, 500, 1000, 1500)

* Unless otherwise indicated, counts are based on average-size servings.

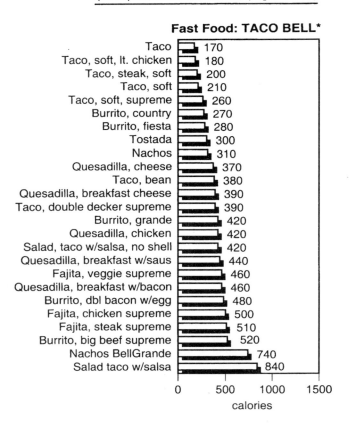

Fast Food: TACO BELL*

Item	calories
Taco	170
Taco, soft, lt. chicken	180
Taco, steak, soft	200
Taco, soft	210
Taco, soft, supreme	260
Burrito, country	270
Burrito, fiesta	280
Tostada	300
Nachos	310
Quesadilla, cheese	370
Taco, bean	380
Quesadilla, breakfast cheese	390
Taco, double decker supreme	390
Burrito, grande	420
Quesadilla, chicken	420
Salad, taco w/salsa, no shell	420
Quesadilla, breakfast w/saus	440
Fajita, veggie supreme	460
Quesadilla, breakfast w/bacon	460
Burrito, dbl bacon w/egg	480
Fajita, chicken supreme	500
Fajita, steak supreme	510
Burrito, big beef supreme	520
Nachos BellGrande	740
Salad taco w/salsa	840

0   500   1000   1500
calories

* Unless otherwise indicated, counts are based on average-
size servings.

Fast Food: WENDY'S*

Item	Calories
Salad, side	60
Hamburger patty, 2 oz	100
Salad, Caesar	100
Chicken only, grilled	110
Salad, garden deluxe	110
Hamburger patty, 1/4 lb	200
Salad, chicken, grilled	200
Taco chips	210
Chicken only, breaded	230
Salad, chicken Caesar	260
Baked potato, plain	310
Sandwich, chicken, grilled	310
Hamburger, plain	360
Baked potato, sour cr & chives	380
Salad, taco	380
Pita, garden, veggie	400
Hamburger, w/everything	420
Sandwich, chicken, breaded	440
Baked potato, broc & cheese	470
Sandwich, chicken club	470
Pita, garden, chicken	480
Baked potato, bacon & cheese	530
Baked potato, cheese	570
Hamburger, bacon classic	580
Baked potato, chili & cheese	630

0   500   1000   1500
calories

* Unless otherwise indicated, counts are based on average-size servings.

Fruits: FRESH & DRIED FRUITS AND JUICES *, Part 1

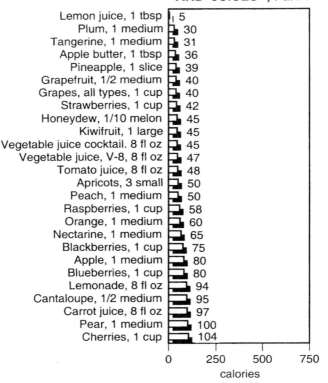

	calories
Lemon juice, 1 tbsp	5
Plum, 1 medium	30
Tangerine, 1 medium	31
Apple butter, 1 tbsp	36
Pineapple, 1 slice	39
Grapefruit, 1/2 medium	40
Grapes, all types, 1 cup	40
Strawberries, 1 cup	42
Honeydew, 1/10 melon	45
Kiwifruit, 1 large	45
Vegetable juice cocktail. 8 fl oz	45
Vegetable juice, V-8, 8 fl oz	47
Tomato juice, 8 fl oz	48
Apricots, 3 small	50
Peach, 1 medium	50
Raspberries, 1 cup	58
Orange, 1 medium	60
Nectarine, 1 medium	65
Blackberries, 1 cup	75
Apple, 1 medium	80
Blueberries, 1 cup	80
Lemonade, 8 fl oz	94
Cantaloupe, 1/2 medium	95
Carrot juice, 8 fl oz	97
Pear, 1 medium	100
Cherries, 1 cup	104

0   250   500   750
calories

* Unless otherwise indicated, counts are based on whole, fresh fruits.

Fruits: FRESH & DRIED FRUITS AND JUICES *, Part 2

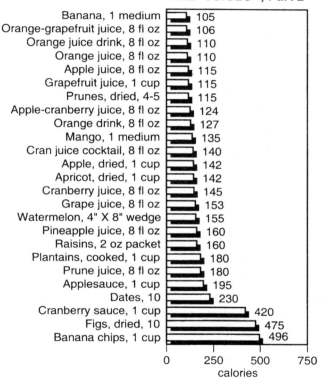

Food	calories
Banana, 1 medium	105
Orange-grapefruit juice, 8 fl oz	106
Orange juice drink, 8 fl oz	110
Orange juice, 8 fl oz	110
Apple juice, 8 fl oz	115
Grapefruit juice, 1 cup	115
Prunes, dried, 4-5	115
Apple-cranberry juice, 8 fl oz	124
Orange drink, 8 fl oz	127
Mango, 1 medium	135
Cran juice cocktail, 8 fl oz	140
Apple, dried, 1 cup	142
Apricot, dried, 1 cup	142
Cranberry juice, 8 fl oz	145
Grape juice, 8 fl oz	153
Watermelon, 4" X 8" wedge	155
Pineapple juice, 8 fl oz	160
Raisins, 2 oz packet	160
Plantains, cooked, 1 cup	180
Prune juice, 8 fl oz	180
Applesauce, 1 cup	195
Dates, 10	230
Cranberry sauce, 1 cup	420
Figs, dried, 10	475
Banana chips, 1 cup	496

* Unless otherwise indicated, counts are based on whole, fresh fruits.

123

GRAVIES, SAUCES & DIPS*

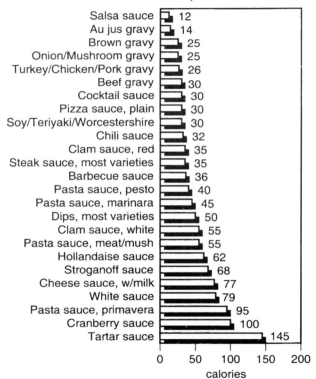

Food	calories
Salsa sauce	12
Au jus gravy	14
Brown gravy	25
Onion/Mushroom gravy	25
Turkey/Chicken/Pork gravy	26
Beef gravy	30
Cocktail sauce	30
Pizza sauce, plain	30
Soy/Teriyaki/Worcestershire	30
Chili sauce	32
Clam sauce, red	35
Steak sauce, most varieties	35
Barbecue sauce	36
Pasta sauce, pesto	40
Pasta sauce, marinara	45
Dips, most varieties	50
Clam sauce, white	55
Pasta sauce, meat/mush	55
Hollandaise sauce	62
Stroganoff sauce	68
Cheese sauce, w/milk	77
White sauce	79
Pasta sauce, primavera	95
Cranberry sauce	100
Tartar sauce	145

calories

* Counts are based on one-quarter cup servings.

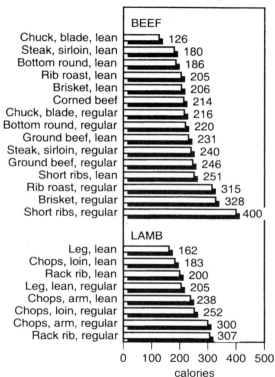

Hi-Low Comparison Chart
(for Alphabetical Charts, see pages 1 - 82)

MEATS*, Part 1

BEEF

Chuck, blade, lean	126
Steak, sirloin, lean	180
Bottom round, lean	186
Rib roast, lean	205
Brisket, lean	206
Corned beef	214
Chuck, blade, regular	216
Bottom round, regular	220
Ground beef, lean	231
Steak, sirloin, regular	240
Ground beef, regular	246
Short ribs, lean	251
Rib roast, regular	315
Brisket, regular	328
Short ribs, regular	400

LAMB

Leg, lean	162
Chops, loin, lean	183
Rack rib, lean	200
Leg, lean, regular	205
Chops, arm, lean	238
Chops, loin, regular	252
Chops, arm, regular	300
Rack rib, regular	307

0   100   200   300   400   500
calories

* Counts are based on 3-ounce servings.

MEATS*, Part 2

LIVER

Liver, chicken, simmered	134
Liver, turkey, simmered	144
Liver, beef, pan-fried	184

PORK

Bacon	105
Bacon, Canadian	105
Ham, cured, lean	131
Chop, lean, broiled	190
Ham, cured, regular	205
Shoulder, lean	206
Chop, regular, broiled	266
Shoulder, regular	295

VEAL

Cutlet, broiled	185
Cutlet, breaded, fried	220
Roasted	230

OTHER MEATS

Venison	134
Rabbit	150
Beefalo	165
Tongue: beef, lamb, pork	234

0   100   200   300   400   500
calories

* Counts are based on 3-ounce servings.

MEATS, PROCESSED*

Item	Calories
Sausage, brown & serve, lean	60
Sausage, brown & serve	70
Beef jerky	90
Chicken breast, sliced	90
Pastrami, turkey	90
Turkey breast/roll, deli style	90
Turkey breast/roll, lean, lite	90
Ham, lite/lean	93
Bacon	105
Bacon, Canadian	105
Chicken roll	105
Corned beef, lite	105
Roast beef, lite/lean	105
Pastrami	120
Roast beef, regular	120
Ham, boiled	150
Salami, turkey	150
Hot dog	180
Sausage, Italian	185
Salami, all beef	210
Corned beef	213
Kielbasa, lite/lean	216
Bologna	255
Kielbasa, regular	285
Salami, dry, hard	360

0   100   200   300   400   500
calories

* Counts are based on 3-ounce servings.

127

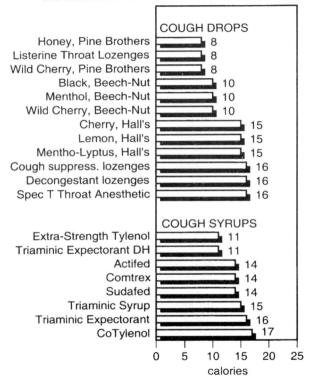

Hi-Low Comparison Chart
(for Alphabetical Charts, see pages 1 - 82)

Medications: COUGH DROPS & SYRUPS*

COUGH DROPS

Honey, Pine Brothers	8
Listerine Throat Lozenges	8
Wild Cherry, Pine Brothers	8
Black, Beech-Nut	10
Menthol, Beech-Nut	10
Wild Cherry, Beech-Nut	10
Cherry, Hall's	15
Lemon, Hall's	15
Mentho-Lyptus, Hall's	15
Cough suppress. lozenges	16
Decongestant lozenges	16
Spec T Throat Anesthetic	16

COUGH SYRUPS

Extra-Strength Tylenol	11
Triaminic Expectorant DH	11
Actifed	14
Comtrex	14
Sudafed	14
Triaminic Syrup	15
Triaminic Expectorant	16
CoTylenol	17

calories
0   5   10   15   20   25

* Counts are based one cough dorop or on recommended
doses for adults.

Medications: OVER-THE-COUNTER REMEDIES & VITAMINS AND MINERALS*

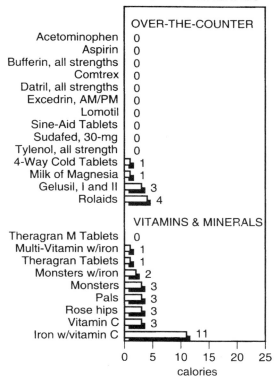

OVER-THE-COUNTER

Acetominophen	0
Aspirin	0
Bufferin, all strengths	0
Comtrex	0
Datril, all strengths	0
Excedrin, AM/PM	0
Lomotil	0
Sine-Aid Tablets	0
Sudafed, 30-mg	0
Tylenol, all strength	0
4-Way Cold Tablets	1
Milk of Magnesia	1
Gelusil, I and II	3
Rolaids	4

VITAMINS & MINERALS

Theragran M Tablets	0
Multi-Vitamin w/iron	1
Theragran Tablets	1
Monsters w/iron	2
Monsters	3
Pals	3
Rose hips	3
Vitamin C	3
Iron w/vitamin C	11

0   5   10   15   20   25
calories

* Counts are based on recommended doses for adults.

MISCELLANEOUS FOODS*

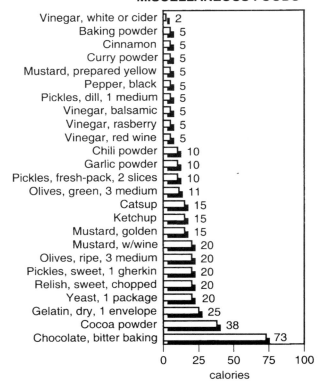

Food	calories
Vinegar, white or cider	2
Baking powder	5
Cinnamon	5
Curry powder	5
Mustard, prepared yellow	5
Pepper, black	5
Pickles, dill, 1 medium	5
Vinegar, balsamic	5
Vinegar, rasberry	5
Vinegar, red wine	5
Chili powder	10
Garlic powder	10
Pickles, fresh-pack, 2 slices	10
Olives, green, 3 medium	11
Catsup	15
Ketchup	15
Mustard, golden	15
Mustard, w/wine	20
Olives, ripe, 3 medium	20
Pickles, sweet, 1 gherkin	20
Relish, sweet, chopped	20
Yeast, 1 package	20
Gelatin, dry, 1 envelope	25
Cocoa powder	38
Chocolate, bitter baking	73

calories

* Unless otherwise indicated, counts are based on
a one-tablespoon serving.

NUTS, BEANS AND SEEDS*: Part #1

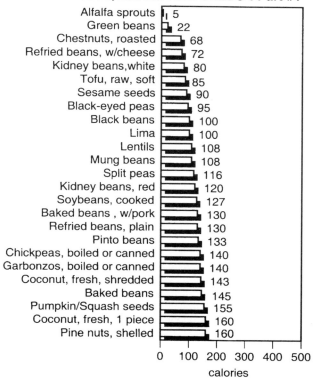

Food	calories
Alfalfa sprouts	5
Green beans	22
Chestnuts, roasted	68
Refried beans, w/cheese	72
Kidney beans, white	80
Tofu, raw, soft	85
Sesame seeds	90
Black-eyed peas	95
Black beans	100
Lima	100
Lentils	108
Mung beans	108
Split peas	116
Kidney beans, red	120
Soybeans, cooked	127
Baked beans , w/pork	130
Refried beans, plain	130
Pinto beans	133
Chickpeas, boiled or canned	140
Garbonzos, boiled or canned	140
Coconut, fresh, shredded	143
Baked beans	145
Pumpkin/Squash seeds	155
Coconut, fresh, 1 piece	160
Pine nuts, shelled	160

0   100   200   300   400   500
calories

* Unless otherwise indicated, counts are based on 1/2 cup
tofu or cooked beans or one-ounce servings of raw nuts or
seeds.

NUTS, BEANS AND SEEDS*: Part #2

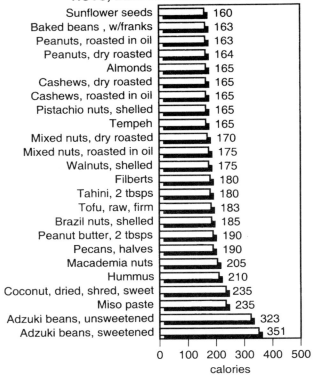

Food	calories
Sunflower seeds	160
Baked beans , w/franks	163
Peanuts, roasted in oil	163
Peanuts, dry roasted	164
Almonds	165
Cashews, dry roasted	165
Cashews, roasted in oil	165
Pistachio nuts, shelled	165
Tempeh	165
Mixed nuts, dry roasted	170
Mixed nuts, roasted in oil	175
Walnuts, shelled	175
Filberts	180
Tahini, 2 tbsps	180
Tofu, raw, firm	183
Brazil nuts, shelled	185
Peanut butter, 2 tbsps	190
Pecans, halves	190
Macadamia nuts	205
Hummus	210
Coconut, dried, shred, sweet	235
Miso paste	235
Adzuki beans, unsweetened	323
Adzuki beans, sweetened	351

calories (0 100 200 300 400 500)

* Unless otherwise indicated, counts are based on 1/2 cup
tofu or cooked beans or one-ounce servings of raw nuts or
seeds.

Hi-Low Comparison Chart
(for Alphabetical Charts, see pages 1 - 82)

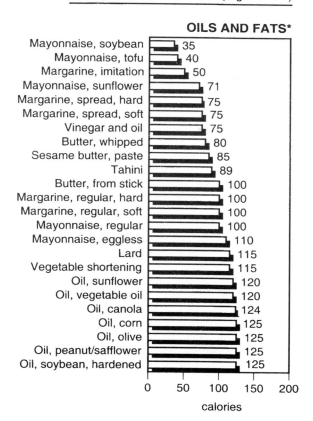

OILS AND FATS*

Food	calories
Mayonnaise, soybean	35
Mayonnaise, tofu	40
Margarine, imitation	50
Mayonnaise, sunflower	71
Margarine, spread, hard	75
Margarine, spread, soft	75
Vinegar and oil	75
Butter, whipped	80
Sesame butter, paste	85
Tahini	89
Butter, from stick	100
Margarine, regular, hard	100
Margarine, regular, soft	100
Mayonnaise, regular	100
Mayonnaise, eggless	110
Lard	115
Vegetable shortening	115
Oil, sunflower	120
Oil, vegetable oil	120
Oil, canola	124
Oil, corn	125
Oil, olive	125
Oil, peanut/safflower	125
Oil, soybean, hardened	125

* Counts are based on 1-tablespoon servings.

PASTA, WHOLE GRAINS , RICE & NOODLES*, Part 1

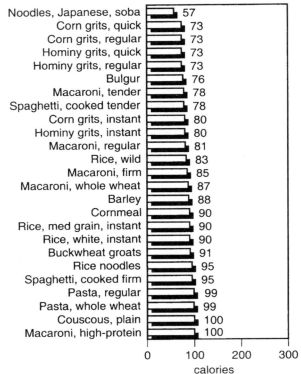

	calories
Noodles, Japanese, soba	57
Corn grits, quick	73
Corn grits, regular	73
Hominy grits, quick	73
Hominy grits, regular	73
Bulgur	76
Macaroni, tender	78
Spaghetti, cooked tender	78
Corn grits, instant	80
Hominy grits, instant	80
Macaroni, regular	81
Rice, wild	83
Macaroni, firm	85
Macaroni, whole wheat	87
Barley	88
Cornmeal	90
Rice, med grain, instant	90
Rice, white, instant	90
Buckwheat groats	91
Rice noodles	95
Spaghetti, cooked firm	95
Pasta, regular	99
Pasta, whole wheat	99
Couscous, plain	100
Macaroni, high-protein	100

* Counts based on cooked, 1/2-cup servings.

PASTA, WHOLE GRAINS , RICE & NOODLES*, Part 2

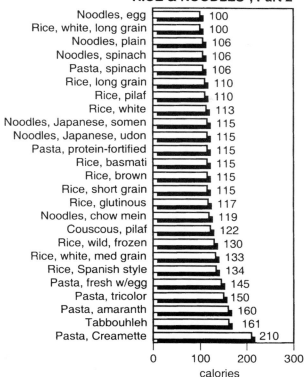

Food	calories
Noodles, egg	100
Rice, white, long grain	100
Noodles, plain	106
Noodles, spinach	106
Pasta, spinach	106
Rice, long grain	110
Rice, pilaf	110
Rice, white	113
Noodles, Japanese, somen	115
Noodles, Japanese, udon	115
Pasta, protein-fortified	115
Rice, basmati	115
Rice, brown	115
Rice, short grain	115
Rice, glutinous	117
Noodles, chow mein	119
Couscous, pilaf	122
Rice, wild, frozen	130
Rice, white, med grain	133
Rice, Spanish style	134
Pasta, fresh w/egg	145
Pasta, tricolor	150
Pasta, amaranth	160
Tabbouhleh	161
Pasta, Creamette	210

* Counts based on cooked, 1/2-cup servings.

Poultry: CHICKEN, TURKEY, AND OTHER FOWL*

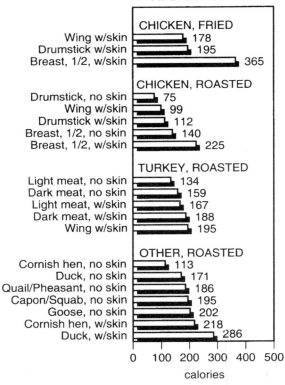

CHICKEN, FRIED

Wing w/skin — 178
Drumstick w/skin — 195
Breast, 1/2, w/skin — 365

CHICKEN, ROASTED

Drumstick, no skin — 75
Wing w/skin — 99
Drumstick w/skin — 112
Breast, 1/2, no skin — 140
Breast, 1/2, w/skin — 225

TURKEY, ROASTED

Light meat, no skin — 134
Dark meat, no skin — 159
Light meat, w/skin — 167
Dark meat, w/skin — 188
Wing w/skin — 195

OTHER, ROASTED

Cornish hen, no skin — 113
Duck, no skin — 171
Quail/Pheasant, no skin — 186
Capon/Squab, no skin — 195
Goose, no skin — 202
Cornish hen, w/skin — 218
Duck, w/skin — 286

0   100 200 300 400 500
calories

* Unless otherwise indicated, counts are based on 3-ounce
servings.

136

SALAD BAR CHOICES*

Food	calories
Alfalfa sprouts	2
Lettuce	2
Cucumber	3
Cabbage	5
Broccoli	6
Cauliflower	6
Green pepper	6
Bean sprouts	8
Carrots	12
Onions, chopped	14
Cantaloupe/Honeydew	15
Beets	18
Croutons	28
Peas	28
Cottage cheese	29
Peaches	48
Gelatin parfait	50
Chickpeas/Garbonzos	55
Chinese noodles	55
Granola	65
Pasta/Macaroni salad	93
Cheddar cheese	100
Egg, chopped	110
Bacon bits	132
Sunflower seeds	160

calories: 0   50   100   150   200

* Counts are based on one-quarter cup servings.

SALAD DRESSINGS*

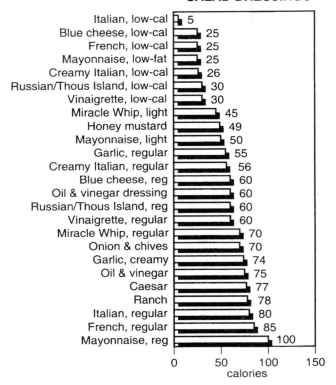

Dressing	calories
Italian, low-cal	5
Blue cheese, low-cal	25
French, low-cal	25
Mayonnaise, low-fat	25
Creamy Italian, low-cal	26
Russian/Thous Island, low-cal	30
Vinaigrette, low-cal	30
Miracle Whip, light	45
Honey mustard	49
Mayonnaise, light	50
Garlic, regular	55
Creamy Italian, regular	56
Blue cheese, reg	60
Oil & vinegar dressing	60
Russian/Thous Island, reg	60
Vinaigrette, regular	60
Miracle Whip, regular	70
Onion & chives	70
Garlic, creamy	74
Oil & vinegar	75
Caesar	77
Ranch	78
Italian, regular	80
French, regular	85
Mayonnaise, reg	100

* For ease of comparison, counts are based on single-tablespoon servings. Adjust counts to reflect quantities consumed.

138

Hi-Low Comparison Chart
(for Alphabetical Charts, see pages 1 - 82)

SEAFOOD*, Part 1

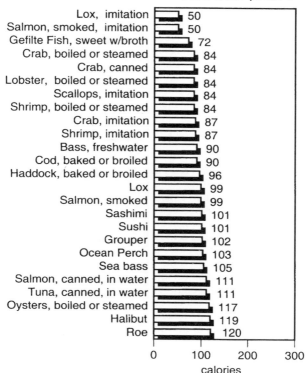

Item	calories
Lox, imitation	50
Salmon, smoked, imitation	50
Gefilte Fish, sweet w/broth	72
Crab, boiled or steamed	84
Crab, canned	84
Lobster, boiled or steamed	84
Scallops, imitation	84
Shrimp, boiled or steamed	84
Crab, imitation	87
Shrimp, imitation	87
Bass, freshwater	90
Cod, baked or broiled	90
Haddock, baked or broiled	96
Lox	99
Salmon, smoked	99
Sashimi	101
Sushi	101
Grouper	102
Ocean Perch	103
Sea bass	105
Salmon, canned, in water	111
Tuna, canned, in water	111
Oysters, boiled or steamed	117
Halibut	119
Roe	120

* Counts are based on 3-ounce servings. Canned seafood
items are assumed to be drained.

139

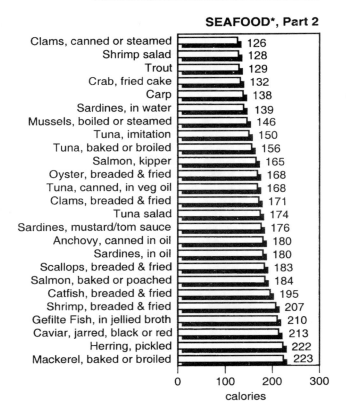

Hi-Low Comparison Chart
(for Alphabetical Charts, see pages 1 - 82)

SEAFOOD*, Part 2

Food	Calories
Clams, canned or steamed	126
Shrimp salad	128
Trout	129
Crab, fried cake	132
Carp	138
Sardines, in water	139
Mussels, boiled or steamed	146
Tuna, imitation	150
Tuna, baked or broiled	156
Salmon, kipper	165
Oyster, breaded & fried	168
Tuna, canned, in veg oil	168
Clams, breaded & fried	171
Tuna salad	174
Sardines, mustard/tom sauce	176
Anchovy, canned in oil	180
Sardines, in oil	180
Scallops, breaded & fried	183
Salmon, baked or poached	184
Catfish, breaded & fried	195
Shrimp, breaded & fried	207
Gefilte Fish, in jellied broth	210
Caviar, jarred, black or red	213
Herring, pickled	222
Mackerel, baked or broiled	223

0   100   200   300
calories

* Counts are based on 3-ounce servings. Canned seafood
items are assumed to be drained.

140

SNACK FOODS AND CHIPS: Part 1*

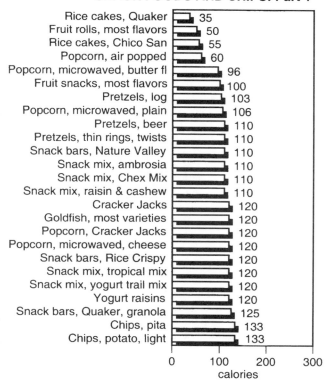

Food	calories
Rice cakes, Quaker	35
Fruit rolls, most flavors	50
Rice cakes, Chico San	55
Popcorn, air popped	60
Popcorn, microwaved, butter fl	96
Fruit snacks, most flavors	100
Pretzels, log	103
Popcorn, microwaved, plain	106
Pretzels, beer	110
Pretzels, thin rings, twists	110
Snack bars, Nature Valley	110
Snack mix, ambrosia	110
Snack mix, Chex Mix	110
Snack mix, raisin & cashew	110
Cracker Jacks	120
Goldfish, most varieties	120
Popcorn, Cracker Jacks	120
Popcorn, microwaved, cheese	120
Snack bars, Rice Crispy	120
Snack mix, tropical mix	120
Snack mix, yogurt trail mix	120
Yogurt raisins	120
Snack bars, Quaker, granola	125
Chips, pita	133
Chips, potato, light	133

* For ease of comparison, counts are based on one-ounce
servings. For popcorn, 1 ounce unpopped = 2 cups popped.
Adjust count to reflect amount consumed.

SNACK FOODS AND CHIPS: Part 2*

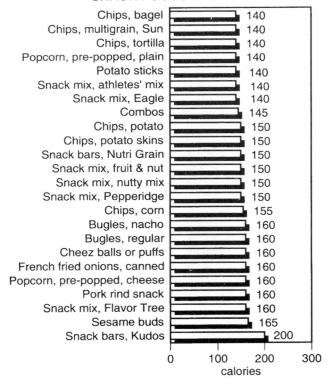

Food	calories
Chips, bagel	140
Chips, multigrain, Sun	140
Chips, tortilla	140
Popcorn, pre-popped, plain	140
Potato sticks	140
Snack mix, athletes' mix	140
Snack mix, Eagle	140
Combos	145
Chips, potato	150
Chips, potato skins	150
Snack bars, Nutri Grain	150
Snack mix, fruit & nut	150
Snack mix, nutty mix	150
Snack mix, Pepperidge	150
Chips, corn	155
Bugles, nacho	160
Bugles, regular	160
Cheez balls or puffs	160
French fried onions, canned	160
Popcorn, pre-popped, cheese	160
Pork rind snack	160
Snack mix, Flavor Tree	160
Sesame buds	165
Snack bars, Kudos	200

* For ease of comparison, counts are based on one-ounce
servings. For popcorn, 1 ounce unpopped = 2 cups popped.
Adjust count to reflect amount consumed.

SOUP, Part 1

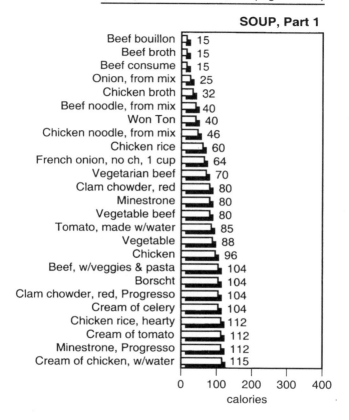

Food	calories
Beef bouillon	15
Beef broth	15
Beef consume	15
Onion, from mix	25
Chicken broth	32
Beef noodle, from mix	40
Won Ton	40
Chicken noodle, from mix	46
Chicken rice	60
French onion, no ch, 1 cup	64
Vegetarian beef	70
Clam chowder, red	80
Minestrone	80
Vegetable beef	80
Tomato, made w/water	85
Vegetable	88
Chicken	96
Beef, w/veggies & pasta	104
Borscht	104
Clam chowder, red, Progresso	104
Cream of celery	104
Chicken rice, hearty	112
Cream of tomato	112
Minestrone, Progresso	112
Cream of chicken, w/water	115

calories (0 100 200 300 400)

* Unless otherwise indicated, counts are based on one-cup
servings.

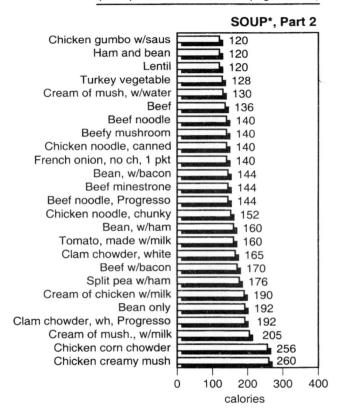

Hi-Low Comparison Chart
(for Alphabetical Charts, see pages 1 - 82)

SOUP*, Part 2

Soup	Calories
Chicken gumbo w/saus	120
Ham and bean	120
Lentil	120
Turkey vegetable	128
Cream of mush, w/water	130
Beef	136
Beef noodle	140
Beefy mushroom	140
Chicken noodle, canned	140
French onion, no ch, 1 pkt	140
Bean, w/bacon	144
Beef minestrone	144
Beef noodle, Progresso	144
Chicken noodle, chunky	152
Bean, w/ham	160
Tomato, made w/milk	160
Clam chowder, white	165
Beef w/bacon	170
Split pea w/ham	176
Cream of chicken w/milk	190
Bean only	192
Clam chowder, wh, Progresso	192
Cream of mush., w/milk	205
Chicken corn chowder	256
Chicken creamy mush	260

calories (0 100 200 300 400)

* Counts are based on one-cup servings.

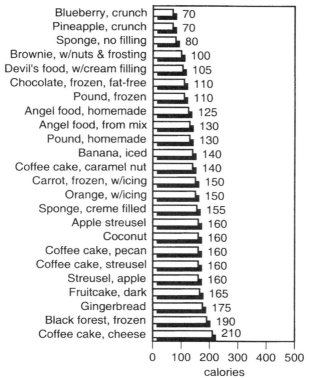

Sweets: CAKES*, Part 1

	calories
Blueberry, crunch	70
Pineapple, crunch	70
Sponge, no filling	80
Brownie, w/nuts & frosting	100
Devil's food, w/cream filling	105
Chocolate, frozen, fat-free	110
Pound, frozen	110
Angel food, homemade	125
Angel food, from mix	130
Pound, homemade	130
Banana, iced	140
Coffee cake, caramel nut	140
Carrot, frozen, w/icing	150
Orange, w/icing	150
Sponge, creme filled	155
Apple streusel	160
Coconut	160
Coffee cake, pecan	160
Coffee cake, streusel	160
Streusel, apple	160
Fruitcake, dark	165
Gingerbread	175
Black forest, frozen	190
Coffee cake, cheese	210

* Counts are based on average-size pieces and slices,
where appropriate, as indicated on package.

145

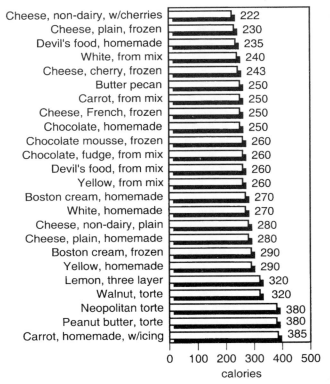

Hi-Low Comparison Chart
(for Alphabetical Charts, see pages 1 - 82)

Sweets: CAKES*, Part 2

	calories
Cheese, non-dairy, w/cherries	222
Cheese, plain, frozen	230
Devil's food, homemade	235
White, from mix	240
Cheese, cherry, frozen	243
Butter pecan	250
Carrot, from mix	250
Cheese, French, frozen	250
Chocolate, homemade	250
Chocolate mousse, frozen	260
Chocolate, fudge, from mix	260
Devil's food, from mix	260
Yellow, from mix	260
Boston cream, homemade	270
White, homemade	270
Cheese, non-dairy, plain	280
Cheese, plain, homemade	280
Boston cream, frozen	290
Yellow, homemade	290
Lemon, three layer	320
Walnut, torte	320
Neopolitan torte	380
Peanut butter, torte	380
Carrot, homemade, w/icing	385

* Counts are based on average-size pieces and slices,
where appropriate, as indicated on package.

146

Sweets: SNACK CAKES*

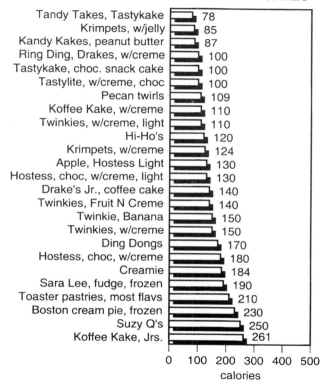

	calories
Tandy Takes, Tastykake	78
Krimpets, w/jelly	85
Kandy Kakes, peanut butter	87
Ring Ding, Drakes, w/creme	100
Tastykake, choc. snack cake	100
Tastylite, w/creme, choc	100
Pecan twirls	109
Koffee Kake, w/creme	110
Twinkies, w/creme, light	110
Hi-Ho's	120
Krimpets, w/creme	124
Apple, Hostess Light	130
Hostess, choc, w/creme, light	130
Drake's Jr., coffee cake	140
Twinkies, Fruit N Creme	140
Twinkie, Banana	150
Twinkies, w/creme	150
Ding Dongs	170
Hostess, choc, w/creme	180
Creamie	184
Sara Lee, fudge, frozen	190
Toaster pastries, most flavs	210
Boston cream pie, frozen	230
Suzy Q's	250
Koffee Kake, Jrs.	261

0   100   200   300   400   500
calories

* Counts are based on average-size pieces and slices,
where appropriate, as indicated on package.

Sweets: CANDY*, Part 1

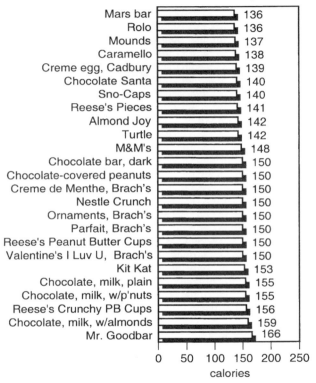

	calories
Mars bar	136
Rolo	136
Mounds	137
Caramello	138
Creme egg, Cadbury	139
Chocolate Santa	140
Sno-Caps	140
Reese's Pieces	141
Almond Joy	142
Turtle	142
M&M's	148
Chocolate bar, dark	150
Chocolate-covered peanuts	150
Creme de Menthe, Brach's	150
Nestle Crunch	150
Ornaments, Brach's	150
Parfait, Brach's	150
Reese's Peanut Butter Cups	150
Valentine's I Luv U, Brach's	150
Kit Kat	153
Chocolate, milk, plain	155
Chocolate, milk, w/p'nuts	155
Reese's Crunchy PB Cups	156
Chocolate, milk, w/almonds	159
Mr. Goodbar	166

* For ease of comparison, counts are based on one-ounce
servings. Adjust counts to reflect quantities consumed.

Sweets: CANDY*, Part 2

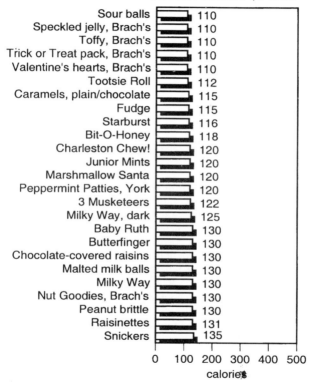

	calories
Sour balls	110
Speckled jelly, Brach's	110
Toffy, Brach's	110
Trick or Treat pack, Brach's	110
Valentine's hearts, Brach's	110
Tootsie Roll	112
Caramels, plain/chocolate	115
Fudge	115
Starburst	116
Bit-O-Honey	118
Charleston Chew!	120
Junior Mints	120
Marshmallow Santa	120
Peppermint Patties, York	120
3 Musketeers	122
Milky Way, dark	125
Baby Ruth	130
Butterfinger	130
Chocolate-covered raisins	130
Malted milk balls	130
Milky Way	130
Nut Goodies, Brach's	130
Peanut brittle	130
Raisinettes	131
Snickers	135

* For ease of comparison, counts are based on one-ounce
servings. Adjust counts to reflect quantities consumed.

Sweets: CANDY*, Part 3

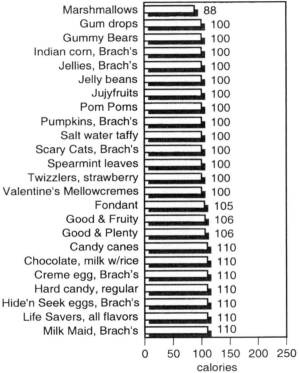

	calories
Marshmallows	88
Gum drops	100
Gummy Bears	100
Indian corn, Brach's	100
Jellies, Brach's	100
Jelly beans	100
Jujyfruits	100
Pom Poms	100
Pumpkins, Brach's	100
Salt water taffy	100
Scary Cats, Brach's	100
Spearmint leaves	100
Twizzlers, strawberry	100
Valentine's Mellowcremes	100
Fondant	105
Good & Fruity	106
Good & Plenty	106
Candy canes	110
Chocolate, milk w/rice	110
Creme egg, Brach's	110
Hard candy, regular	110
Hide'n Seek eggs, Brach's	110
Life Savers, all flavors	110
Milk Maid, Brach's	110

*   For ease of comparison, counts are based on one-ounce
    servings. Adjust counts to reflect quantities consumed.

Sweets: COOKIES*, Part 1

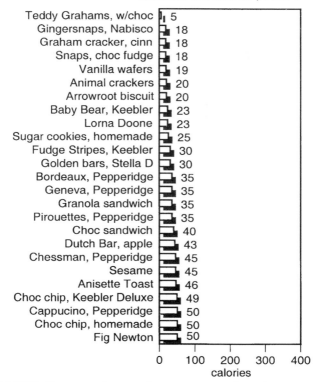

	calories
Teddy Grahams, w/choc	5
Gingersnaps, Nabisco	18
Graham cracker, cinn	18
Snaps, choc fudge	18
Vanilla wafers	19
Animal crackers	20
Arrowroot biscuit	20
Baby Bear, Keebler	23
Lorna Doone	23
Sugar cookies, homemade	25
Fudge Stripes, Keebler	30
Golden bars, Stella D	30
Bordeaux, Pepperidge	35
Geneva, Pepperidge	35
Granola sandwich	35
Pirouettes, Pepperidge	35
Choc sandwich	40
Dutch Bar, apple	43
Chessman, Pepperidge	45
Sesame	45
Anisette Toast	46
Choc chip, Keebler Deluxe	49
Cappucino, Pepperidge	50
Choc chip, homemade	50
Fig Newton	50

0   100   200   300   400
calories

* NOTE: For ease of comparison, counts are based on
single cookie servings. When more than one cookie is
consumed, counts should be adjusted accordingly.

Sweets: COOKIES*, Part 2

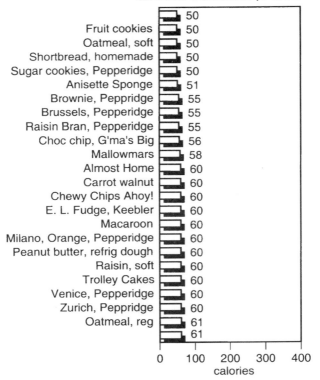

	calories
	50
Fruit cookies	50
Oatmeal, soft	50
Shortbread, homemade	50
Sugar cookies, Pepperidge	50
Anisette Sponge	51
Brownie, Peppridge	55
Brussels, Pepperidge	55
Raisin Bran, Pepperidge	55
Choc chip, G'ma's Big	56
Mallowmars	58
Almost Home	60
Carrot walnut	60
Chewy Chips Ahoy!	60
E. L. Fudge, Keebler	60
Macaroon	60
Milano, Orange, Pepperidge	60
Peanut butter, refrig dough	60
Raisin, soft	60
Trolley Cakes	60
Venice, Pepperidge	60
Zurich, Peppridge	60
Oatmeal, reg	61
	61

* NOTE: For ease of comparison, counts are based on
single cookie servings. When more than one cookie is
consumed, counts should be adjusted accordingly.

152

Sweets: COOKIES*, Part 3

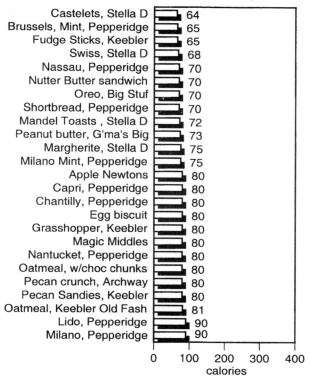

	calories
Castelets, Stella D	64
Brussels, Mint, Pepperidge	65
Fudge Sticks, Keebler	65
Swiss, Stella D	68
Nassau, Pepperidge	70
Nutter Butter sandwich	70
Oreo, Big Stuf	70
Shortbread, Pepperidge	70
Mandel Toasts , Stella D	72
Peanut butter, G'ma's Big	73
Margherite, Stella D	75
Milano Mint, Pepperidge	75
Apple Newtons	80
Capri, Pepperidge	80
Chantilly, Pepperidge	80
Egg biscuit	80
Grasshopper, Keebler	80
Magic Middles	80
Nantucket, Pepperidge	80
Oatmeal, w/choc chunks	80
Pecan crunch, Archway	80
Pecan Sandies, Keebler	80
Oatmeal, Keebler Old Fash	81
Lido, Pepperidge	90
Milano, Pepperidge	90

0   100   200   300   400
calories

* NOTE: For ease of comparison, counts are based on
single cookie servings. When more than one cookie is
consumed, counts should be adjusted accordingly.

Sweets: COOKIES*, Part 4

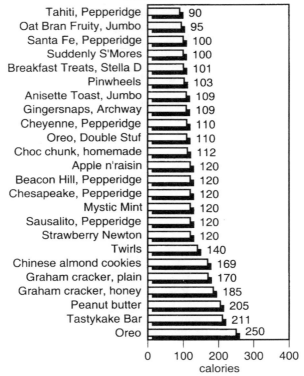

Cookie	calories
Tahiti, Pepperidge	90
Oat Bran Fruity, Jumbo	95
Santa Fe, Pepperidge	100
Suddenly S'Mores	100
Breakfast Treats, Stella D	101
Pinwheels	103
Anisette Toast, Jumbo	109
Gingersnaps, Archway	109
Cheyenne, Pepperidge	110
Oreo, Double Stuf	110
Choc chunk, homemade	112
Apple n'raisin	120
Beacon Hill, Pepperidge	120
Chesapeake, Pepperidge	120
Mystic Mint	120
Sausalito, Pepperidge	120
Strawberry Newton	120
Twirls	140
Chinese almond cookies	169
Graham cracker, plain	170
Graham cracker, honey	185
Peanut butter	205
Tastykake Bar	211
Oreo	250

0   100   200   300   400
calories

* NOTE: For ease of comparison, counts are based on
single cookie servings. When more than one cookie is
consumed, counts should be adjusted accordingly.

154

Sweets: DONUTS*

Donut	Calories
Glazed, plain	180
Lemon	200
Filled, Bavarian cream	210
Filled, black raspberry	210
Filled, jelly	210
Frosted, van/straw icing	210
Cruller, plain	240
Filled, Boston cream	240
Cruller, sugar	250
Plain, cake	250
Sugared	250
Cinnamon	270
Cruller, powdered	270
Eclair	270
Filled, chocolate cream	270
Filled, vanilla cream	270
Powdered	270
Cruller, glazed, chocolate	280
Cruller, glazed, vanilla	290
Glazed, chocolate, cake	290
Jelly stick	290
Apple fritter	300
Coconut, toasted	300
Frosted, chocolate icing	300
Glazed, whole wheat, cake	310

0   100   200   300   400   500
calories

* Counts are based on average-size donuts.

Sweets: GUM & MINTS*

GUM

	calories
Dentyne, sugarless	5
Beechies	6
Chiclets	6
Dentyne	6
Care Free	8
Chewels	8
Beech-Nut	10
Big Red	10
Bubble Care Free	10
Doublemint	10
Freedent	10
Juicy Fruit	10
Wrigley's Spearmint	10
Freshen-Up	13
Hubba Bubba	23
Bubble Yum	25
Bubblicious	25

MINTS

	calories
Tic Tac	2
Chlorets	6
Breathsavers, spearmint	8

0   10   20   30   40
calories

* Counts are based on single sticks or mints.

156

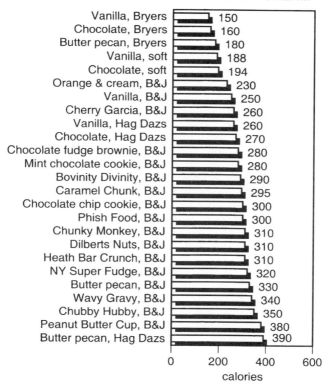

Hi-Low Comparison Chart
(for Alphabetical Charts, see pages 1 - 82)

Sweets: ICE CREAM*

Item	calories
Vanilla, Bryers	150
Chocolate, Bryers	160
Butter pecan, Bryers	180
Vanilla, soft	188
Chocolate, soft	194
Orange & cream, B&J	230
Vanilla, B&J	250
Cherry Garcia, B&J	260
Vanilla, Hag Dazs	260
Chocolate, Hag Dazs	270
Chocolate fudge brownie, B&J	280
Mint chocolate cookie, B&J	280
Bovinity Divinity, B&J	290
Caramel Chunk, B&J	295
Chocolate chip cookie, B&J	300
Phish Food, B&J	300
Chunky Monkey, B&J	310
Dilberts Nuts, B&J	310
Heath Bar Crunch, B&J	310
NY Super Fudge, B&J	320
Butter pecan, B&J	330
Wavy Gravy, B&J	340
Chubby Hubby, B&J	350
Peanut Butter Cup, B&J	380
Butter pecan, Hag Dazs	390

calories (0, 200, 400, 600)

* Counts are based on one-half cup servings. "B&J" designates Ben & Jerry's brand.

Sweets: ICE CREAM CONES & BARS, ICE CREAM ALTERNATIVES AND PUDDINGS*

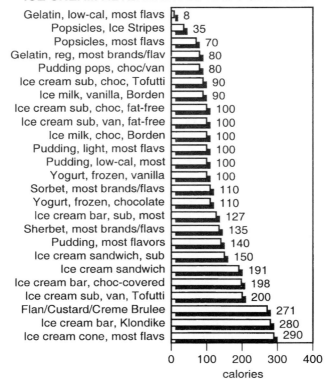

	calories
Gelatin, low-cal, most flavs	8
Popsicles, Ice Stripes	35
Popsicles, most flavs	70
Gelatin, reg, most brands/flav	80
Pudding pops, choc/van	80
Ice cream sub, choc, Tofutti	90
Ice milk, vanilla, Borden	90
Ice cream sub, choc, fat-free	100
Ice cream sub, van, fat-free	100
Ice milk, choc, Borden	100
Pudding, light, most flavs	100
Pudding, low-cal, most	100
Yogurt, frozen, vanilla	100
Sorbet, most brands/flavs	110
Yogurt, frozen, chocolate	110
Ice cream bar, sub, most	127
Sherbet, most brands/flavs	135
Pudding, most flavors	140
Ice cream sandwich, sub	150
Ice cream sandwich	191
Ice cream bar, choc-covered	198
Ice cream sub, van, Tofutti	200
Flan/Custard/Creme Brulee	271
Ice cream bar, Klondike	280
Ice cream cone, most flavs	290

* Counts are based on average- or one-half cup serving.
"Sub" designates non-dairy, ice cream substitute.

158

Sweets: PIES*

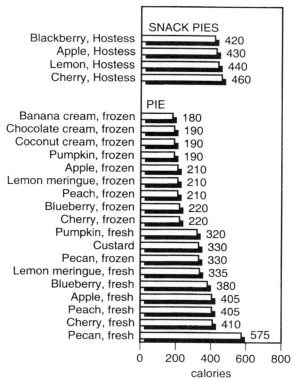

SNACK PIES

	calories
Blackberry, Hostess	420
Apple, Hostess	430
Lemon, Hostess	440
Cherry, Hostess	460

PIE

	calories
Banana cream, frozen	180
Chocolate cream, frozen	190
Coconut cream, frozen	190
Pumpkin, frozen	190
Apple, frozen	210
Lemon meringue, frozen	210
Peach, frozen	210
Blueberry, frozen	220
Cherry, frozen	220
Pumpkin, fresh	320
Custard	330
Pecan, frozen	330
Lemon meringue, fresh	335
Blueberry, fresh	380
Apple, fresh	405
Peach, fresh	405
Cherry, fresh	410
Pecan, fresh	575

0   200   400   600   800
calories

* Counts are based on average-size pieces and slices,
where appropriate, as indicated on package.

Sweets: SUGARS, SYRUPS, TOPPINGS AND JAMS*

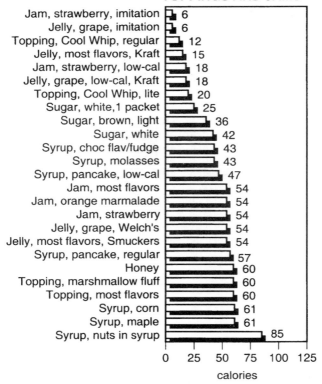

	calories
Jam, strawberry, imitation	6
Jelly, grape, imitation	6
Topping, Cool Whip, regular	12
Jelly, most flavors, Kraft	15
Jam, strawberry, low-cal	18
Jelly, grape, low-cal, Kraft	18
Topping, Cool Whip, lite	20
Sugar, white, 1 packet	25
Sugar, brown, light	36
Sugar, white	42
Syrup, choc flav/fudge	43
Syrup, molasses	43
Syrup, pancake, low-cal	47
Jam, most flavors	54
Jam, orange marmalade	54
Jam, strawberry	54
Jelly, grape, Welch's	54
Jelly, most flavors, Smuckers	54
Syrup, pancake, regular	57
Honey	60
Topping, marshmallow fluff	60
Topping, most flavors	60
Syrup, corn	61
Syrup, maple	61
Syrup, nuts in syrup	85

* Counts are based on single-tablespoon servings. Jams and preserves can be assumed to have equal values.

VEGETABLES*, Part 1

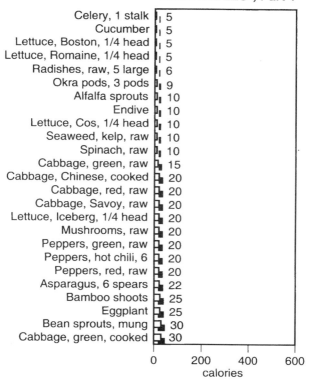

	calories
Celery, 1 stalk	5
Cucumber	5
Lettuce, Boston, 1/4 head	5
Lettuce, Romaine, 1/4 head	5
Radishes, raw, 5 large	6
Okra pods, 3 pods	9
Alfalfa sprouts	10
Endive	10
Lettuce, Cos, 1/4 head	10
Seaweed, kelp, raw	10
Spinach, raw	10
Cabbage, green, raw	15
Cabbage, Chinese, cooked	20
Cabbage, red, raw	20
Cabbage, Savoy, raw	20
Lettuce, Iceberg, 1/4 head	20
Mushrooms, raw	20
Peppers, green, raw	20
Peppers, hot chili, 6	20
Peppers, red, raw	20
Asparagus, 6 spears	22
Bamboo shoots	25
Eggplant	25
Bean sprouts, mung	30
Cabbage, green, cooked	30

calories: 0   200   400   600

* Unless otherwise indicated, counts are based on one-cup
servings. For vegetable juices, see the Fruits & Juices
section.

VEGETABLES*, Part 2

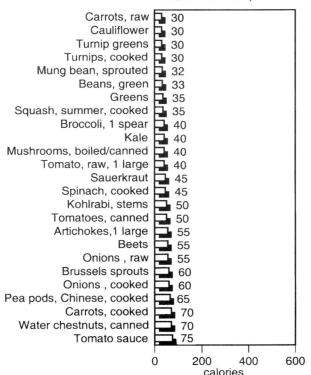

Vegetable	calories
Carrots, raw	30
Cauliflower	30
Turnip greens	30
Turnips, cooked	30
Mung bean, sprouted	32
Beans, green	33
Greens	35
Squash, summer, cooked	35
Broccoli, 1 spear	40
Kale	40
Mushrooms, boiled/canned	40
Tomato, raw, 1 large	40
Sauerkraut	45
Spinach, cooked	45
Kohlrabi, stems	50
Tomatoes, canned	50
Artichokes,1 large	55
Beets	55
Onions , raw	55
Brussels sprouts	60
Onions , cooked	60
Pea pods, Chinese, cooked	65
Carrots, cooked	70
Water chestnuts, canned	70
Tomato sauce	75

0   200   400   600
calories

* Unless otherwise indicated, counts are based on one-cup servings. For vegetable juices, see the Fruits & Juices section.

Hi-Low Comparison Chart
(for Alphabetical Charts, see pages 1 - 82)

VEGETABLES*, Part 3

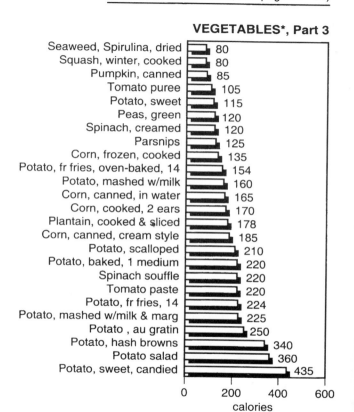

Item	calories
Seaweed, Spirulina, dried	80
Squash, winter, cooked	80
Pumpkin, canned	85
Tomato puree	105
Potato, sweet	115
Peas, green	120
Spinach, creamed	120
Parsnips	125
Corn, frozen, cooked	135
Potato, fr fries, oven-baked, 14	154
Potato, mashed w/milk	160
Corn, canned, in water	165
Corn, cooked, 2 ears	170
Plantain, cooked & sliced	178
Corn, canned, cream style	185
Potato, scalloped	210
Potato, baked, 1 medium	220
Spinach souffle	220
Tomato paste	220
Potato, fr fries, 14	224
Potato, mashed w/milk & marg	225
Potato , au gratin	250
Potato, hash browns	340
Potato salad	360
Potato, sweet, candied	435

* Unless otherwise indicated, counts are based on one-cup servings. For vegetable juices, see the Fruits & Juices section.

VEGETARIAN CHOICES*

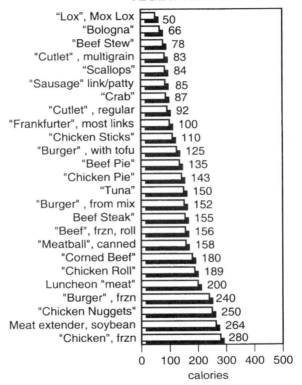

Food	calories
"Lox", Mox Lox	50
"Bologna"	66
"Beef Stew"	78
"Cutlet" , multigrain	83
"Scallops"	84
"Sausage" link/patty	85
"Crab"	87
"Cutlet" , regular	92
"Frankfurter", most links	100
"Chicken Sticks"	110
"Burger" , with tofu	125
"Beef Pie"	135
"Chicken Pie"	143
"Tuna"	150
"Burger" , from mix	152
Beef Steak"	155
"Beef", frzn, roll	156
"Meatball", canned	158
"Corned Beef"	180
"Chicken Roll"	189
Luncheon "meat"	200
"Burger" , frzn	240
"Chicken Nuggets"	250
Meat extender, soybean	264
"Chicken", frzn	280

0 100 200 300 400 500
calories

* Made from tofu, textured vegetable protein or a combination of both. Counts are based on 3-ounce servings.

PLUME

From Drs. Richard F. and Rachael F. Heller

THE CARBOHYDRATE ADDICT'S LIFESPAN PROGRAM
The phenomenal weight-loss program that teaches you how to break your addiction to carbohydrates while enjoying food as you never have before.

0-452-27838-4

**THE CARBOHYDRATE ADDICT'S PROGRAM
FOR SUCCESS**
The companion workbook to *The Carbohydrate Addict's LifeSpan Program*, this essential volume provides additional tools, resources, and support for carbohydrate addicts using this breakthrough program.

0-452-26933-4

HEALTHY FOR LIFE
Reduce your risk of heart disease, diabetes, stroke, cancer, and high blood pressure—without deprivation or sacrifice—through this revolutionary nutritional program designed for lifetime success.

0-452-27112-6
